Quinine

and

QUARANTINE

PROJECT SPONSORS

Missouri Center for the Book

Warren and Clara Cole Estate

**Western Historical Manuscript Collection,
University of Missouri–Columbia**

CONSULTANT

William Crowley, M.D.

SPECIAL THANKS

H. Denny Donnell, M.D.

Fae Sotham, State Historical Society of Missouri, Columbia

MISSOURI HERITAGE READERS

GENERAL EDITOR,

Rebecca B. Schroeder

Each Missouri Heritage Reader explores a particular aspect of the state's rich cultural heritage. Focusing on people, places, historical events, and the details of daily life, these books illustrate the ways in which people from all parts of the world contributed to the development of the state and the region. The books incorporate documentary and oral history, folklore, and informal literature in a way that makes these resources accessible to all Missourians.

Intended primarily for adult new readers, these books will also be invaluable to readers of all ages interested in the cultural and social history of Missouri.

Quinine

and

QUARANTINE

Missouri Medicine through the Years

Loren Humphrey

University of Missouri Press

COLUMBIA AND LONDON

Library of Congress Cataloging-in-Publication Data

Humphrey, Loren, 1931–
   Quinine and quarantine : Missouri medicine through the
years / Loren Humphrey.
      p.   cm. — (Missouri heritage readers)
   Includes bibliographical references and index.
   ISBN 0-8261-1269-7 (alk. paper)
   1. Medicine—Missouri—History. 2. Medical care—
Missouri—History. I. Title. II. Series.

R263.H86 2000
610'.9778—dc21
                                                99-054575

Designer: Elizabeth K. Young
Typesetter: Crane Composition, Inc.
Printer and binder: Thomson-Shore, Inc.
Typefaces: Times New Roman, Academy Engraved

Dedicated to

state and county health officials, past and present,
nurse and physician pioneers, 1799–1998,
the Missouri State Medical Association,
the Missouri Nurses Association, and
to Missourians of the future who continue the
battle to obtain the best possible health for all citizens.

Contents

Acknowledgments

Missourians, those who still live in the state as well as those who have gone elsewhere, have played an important role in bringing the following pages to life. Special thanks go to them for giving their time and sharing personal experiences and thoughts.

The personnel in the State Historical Society of Missouri, Columbia, were of great assistance in digging into the hidden corners of Missouri medicine.

The staff of Archives and Rare Books of Bernard Becker Medical Library of Washington University School of Medicine gave of their time and located resource material.

Dr. William Crowley deserves a special thanks for struggling with me on medical matters, especially for the last period. We sometimes had great difficulty in maintaining perspective for the picture because we were in the frame.

Wendy Evans and Dr. Everett Sugarbaker supplied important data regarding Ellis Fischel. Dr. Frank Mitchell provided details of the trauma system for the state. Dr. E. Grey Dimond was a wonderful help with the Medical School at the University of Missouri, Kansas City, and C. Rollins Hanlon shared many views of medicine in St. Louis and insights into the big American medical picture.

Thank you all for making the task easier—and more fun.

Quinine

and

QUARANTINE

Introduction

Disease was permitted to run its course after the list of family remedies had been exhausted.

—Dr. E. J. Goodwin, *A History of Medicine in Missouri,*
describing medical treatment in Ste. Genevieve in 1793

Medicine is the art or science of preventing disease or injury, when possible, and of restoring health when illness or injury have already occurred. Healing involves correcting mental problems or physical ailments, using drugs and surgical operations, or replacing diseased and worn-out body parts. For Missouri's pioneers, the first aspect, preserving health, was something over which they had some control. The second, restoring health, depended on home remedies or was in the hands of the few physicians to be found in Missouri. They seldom had the knowledge necessary to restore health to the seriously ill or injured.

Health, the absence of illness or physical disorders, depends on favorable environmental factors, absence of inherited defects, and freedom from disease. Missouri's founding fathers recognized the importance of health with the state motto: *Salus populi suprema lex esto* (Let the welfare of the people be the supreme law). By incorporating their concern for the well-being of the state's citizens into the great seal, the founding fathers of Missouri announced to the world that, by law, health takes high priority.

This account considers the two aspects of medicine affecting the well-being of Missourians. County officers who carry out health laws and governmental regulations effect the first, preservation of health, through community activities. Informing the public about environmental risk factors and contagious diseases is their responsibility. Other agencies monitor the number of accidents on public roads or in the workplace and search for ways to make those places safer. Still others monitor ground, water, or air pollu-

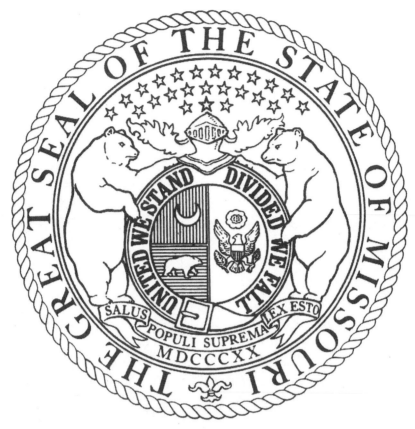

The Great Seal of the State of Missouri has the state motto: SALUS POPULI SUPREMA LEX ESTO (Let the welfare of the people be the supreme law). This Latin expression honors the Roman goddess of health. (State Historical Society of Missouri, Columbia)

tion. County health clinics commonly oversee immunization against polio, childhood diseases, influenza, and impending epidemics. Public health officers are responsible for reporting cases of contagious diseases, including social diseases, and screening for cervical cancer, often in collaboration with local doctors.

Unnoticed at times, the public health worker struggles to improve health for all citizens. In the past, county health workers identified and corrected waste disposal or water supply problems that caused disease, sometimes of epidemic proportions, and posted notices of quarantine when disease struck.

Those city and county health-care workers who pushed the medical profession, educated the public, tested those without access to or the means to afford private care, and at the same time worked with medical professionals have not received Nobel Prizes or other honors. In fact, many are unknown, and their contributions cannot be determined or recognized today.

The medical profession effects the second aspect of medicine: the diagnosis and treatment of diseases and the care of injuries. To carry out this function, physicians, after four years of college, attend medical school for four years. Then they train from three to seven years in specialty residency. Nurses spend five years in training for degrees, and many then spend from two to seven years obtaining advanced degrees to work in special fields of nursing.

To appreciate the status of medicine in Missouri at the end of the twentieth century, its marvels and its challenges, the problems faced and the progress made from Missouri's earliest days to the present must be understood. The history of medicine in Missouri cannot be separated from the general history of the state's development.

The people of Missouri have wrestled with a changing environment, a growing population, and advances in medical knowledge in an attempt to enjoy health. The living conditions during different periods were as important as the treatments offered by the medical profession.

Today the quality of health care in the U.S. is frequently measured by birth mortality (the number of deaths per hundred thousand births) compared with that of other countries. Unfortunately, the United States ranks below many other industrial countries in birth mortality. But this is not as much a measure of health care as it is a reflection of social factors that affect access to medical treatment and contribute to birth mortality. Poverty, poor education, and even transportation are problems for expectant mothers in large cities and rural areas alike. These same factors influence the health of mother and child after birth.

For everyone, environmental factors can contribute to farm,

home, and transportation accidents. Similarly, air and water quality, whether contaminated from industrial waste or human waste, cause health problems. Social problems like substandard education and economic deprivation likewise contribute more to poor health than the absence of medical professionals or inferior care by nurse, physician, or hospital. Hence, as Missouri improved the quality of care given by the medical profession and hospitals through appropriate regulations, efforts were made to educate patients about health and improve access for all citizens to health care.

Up until the early 1800s, Missouri (then Upper Louisiana) had few hospitals or physicians, a sparse population, and practically no newspapers or official records of medical history. Even after Louis Joliet and Father Jacques Marquette explored the Mississippi River as far as present-day Arkansas in 1673, travel was limited, restricting the spread of contagious diseases to early explorers. Threats to the health of the Native American tribes were severe however.

In the early 1700s, the French continued to explore the Missouri River. The Missouri Indians became their allies in war and fur trading. In 1723 the French built a military post named Fort Orleans north of the Missouri River in present-day Carroll County. Historians believe the French colonists established the first permanent settlement on the west bank of the upper Mississippi at Ste. Genevieve about 1750. The area was still called the "Illinois country," and the seat of government was in faraway New Orleans. Local laws prevailed, and concern for health care appears to have been nonexistent. From all indications, physicians assigned to the French military post adjoining the settlement did not make themselves available to the community, so Ste. Genevieve was without a physician until Dr. Bernard Gibkins, a German physician, arrived in the mid–1770s. In *Colonial Ste. Genevieve* Carl J. Ekberg reports that Dr. Gibkins's patients complained about his large bills and the numerous medicines he prescribed, but he practiced in the Ste. Genevieve area until his death in 1783.

In 1764 Pierre Laclede settled at the site that would become St. Louis. By 1770 the settlement had a population of "a few hun-

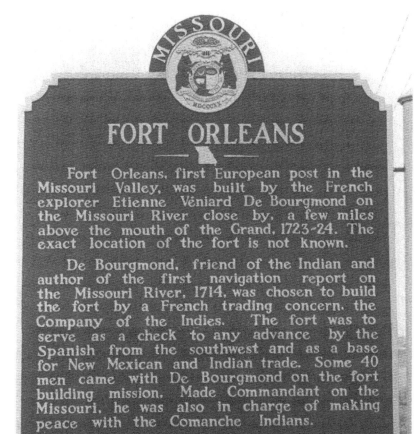

FORT ORLEANS

Fort Orleans, first European post in the Missouri Valley, was built by the French explorer Etienne Véniard De Bourgmond on the Missouri River close by, a few miles above the mouth of the Grand, 1723-24. The exact location of the fort is not known.

De Bourgmond, friend of the Indian and author of the first navigation report on the Missouri River, 1714, was chosen to build the fort by a French trading concern, the Company of the Indies. The fort was to serve as a check to any advance by the Spanish from the southwest and as a base for New Mexican and Indian trade. Some 40 men came with De Bourgmond on the fort building mission. Made Commandant on the Missouri, he was also in charge of making peace with the Comanche Indians.

A village of Missouri Indians was across the river from the fort. These Indians, of Souian stock, at one time called themselves Niutachis. They were probably first called Missouris, Algonquin for "he of the big canoe" by the Illinois Indians. The last of the Missouris died on the Oto Reservation in Oklahoma, 1907.

(See other side)
Erected by State Historical Society of Missouri and State Highway Commission. 1933

Marker for Fort Orleans. The Missouri Indians were devastated by their friendship with the French. They lacked natural resistance to the white man's diseases, such as smallpox, and many died. By the mid–1700s their numbers had been greatly reduced. (photo courtesy A. E. Schroeder)

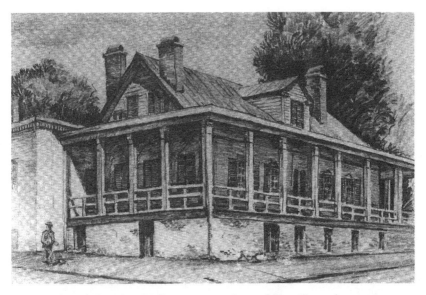

Home of Jean Baptiste Valle, commandant of Ste. Genevieve, who took command of the post in March 1804, as the Americans took over the government of the Louisiana Territory. Soon afterward, he ordered the flag lowered and the "Stars and Stripes" raised. His home is now a State Historic Site. (State Historical Society of Missouri, Columbia)

dred." Dr. Andre Auguste Conde was one of the military surgeons assigned to the military post and was probably the first physician to practice medicine outside a post anywhere in Upper Louisiana. Conde, a native of Annis, France, arrived in St. Louis with his wife and infant daughter. He settled in the new village and practiced there until his death in 1776.

That year, Dr. Antoine Reynal arrived in St. Louis. He practiced in St. Louis and St. Charles for the next twenty-three years. Two years after his arrival, officials made several attempts to improve the sewage and water systems in St. Louis. Unfortunately, their efforts failed. In the years to come, many of the city's citizens would pay the price of this failure: poor health and early death. With the slow communication at the time, the New World, at least along the Mississippi River, seemed ignorant of a new, very contagious disease—cholera. A scourge that came from bacteria that grew in poor sewage and water systems, the disease began in Asia and had reached Missouri by the 1830s.

About seventy colonists recruited by Col. George Morgan had settled at New Madrid, opposite the mouth of the Ohio River, by 1789. At the same time, pioneers from the eastern states were pushing ever farther west along the Missouri River, especially toward present-day Howard County.

Before the nineteenth century, the few settlers west of the Mississippi in Upper Louisiana had to concern themselves with the struggle for existence in an undeveloped environment. Surviving the harsh winters and producing a living from the land preoccupied them. On the whole, Native Americans were friendly, although bands would attack settlers on occasion. During the Revolutionary War, both the British and Americans had Indian allies, and in 1780, some Native Americans attacked Fort St. Louis. The Missouri tribe, which for years had been friendly with the French, was less so with the Spanish or the American pioneers pushing for more land to settle. When their numbers decreased, many of the Missouri joined other tribes, the Iowans, the Otos, and the Kansa, tribes closely related to theirs. The Osage remained until 1825, when they agreed to cede their lands in Missouri and the Arkansas Territory to the United States.

From their contact with Native Americans, pioneers learned to use the surrounding materials, especially herbs and plants, as medicines. With no physicians or pharmacies, settlers relied on medicinal plants as the only resource to combat disease or manage injuries. Pioneers adopted several home remedies from the Missouri and Osage. The Cherokee, who traveled the "Trail of Tears" across Missouri, brought many remedies. One of the missionaries traveling with the Cherokee credited a "healing drink" of slippery-elm tea with curing him and his wife of sickness. For a leg ulcer, Indians used an extract of sassafras bark to bathe the sore, then applied a poultice of powdered maize and turkey down.

Witch hazel, known also as spotted alder, was a crooked tree or shrub that grew from eight to fifteen feet tall. Indians applied the witch hazel's bark to skin for inflammations, and they used the inner bark as a poultice for irritated eyes and chewed it to freshen the mouth. Beech or stone beech, a tree that grew to one hundred feet in height, had silky leaves that were two to five inches long. Both the bark and leaves were useful. After steeping a handful of fresh bark in a cup of water, the Indians used the liquid to treat rashes, especially those from poison ivy. Pioneers learned to make a concoction of fresh leaves, which they applied to burns, scalds, and frostbite.

Showy milkweed, a plant that grew five feet high, had numerous uses; settlers used its milky latex as an antiseptic for ringworm, cuts, and sores and made a tea with it to treat measles, coughs, and tuberculosis. Indian women used the latex on sore breasts. Powdered dried roots of the spotted geranium stopped bleeding from cuts, scratches, and wounds. A variety of other plants provided relief from common ailments. By the time physicians arrived in the early nineteenth century, many treatments had become established as folk medicine, handed down from generation to generation. Others had been adopted as remedies by the medical profession.

Throughout early history, the absence of drugs for relief from pain was a major health problem, an obstacle to surgical treatments and care of the severely injured. Before 1799, Indians and settlers used various concoctions made from plants, such as oil of wintergreen leaves, which contain methylsalicylate, for the aches and pains of rheumatism, childbirth, menstruation, and mild flu-like ailments. Early settlers also commonly relied on whiskey for pain relief.

According to Mike Gruendler, Sharon Matlock, and Carole Mushkin, the inhalation of smoke from the burned tops of purple coneflower gave relief from headache. In the 1988 *Missouri Folklore Society Journal,* which explores uses of wild plants in Missouri, they also reported that Missourians used jack-in-the-pulpit for headache. Settlers pulverized the dried corn and rubbed the dust onto the area affected. The authors list other medicinal plants in Missouri and describe their uses. The issue also contains a section titled "Traditional Uses of Wild Plants in Missouri." Ginny Wallace and Leonard Blake tell how the Osage Indians used native plants for food and for making rope, twine, mats, and many other household items.

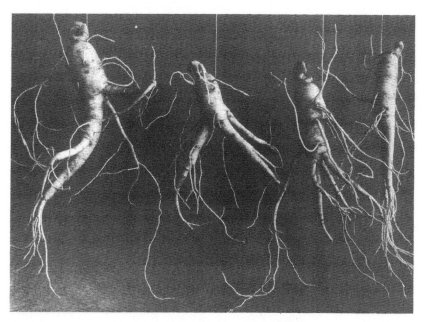

Ginseng root was used as an aphrodisiac and fertility drug by the Chinese. The root of this foot-high, green plant also became popular with the settlers because it increased energy and gave one a sense of general well-being. (State Historical Society of Missouri, Columbia)

In 1775 an English herb doctor, William Withering of Staffordshire, discovered that digitalis, the active ingredient of foxglove (*Digitalis purpurea*), a plant with a drooping, tubular, purple or white flower, could improve cardiac health. Pioneers brought the drug to the frontier and used it for heart problems.

Settlers used ginseng (*Panex quinquefolus L.*), a plant still found in the Ozarks, as a panacea. Mostly it gave a feeling of well-being and soothed an upset stomach, but many people also used it as an aphrodisiac. The Chinese named ginseng ("man plant") for the shape of the mature fork-shaped root: it resembles a man's body.

Today, commercial growers provide both digitalis and ginseng for use by a major pharmaceutical house in Pennsylvania. The fact that Missourians relied on these drugs well into the twentieth century is proof of their effectiveness. Recognition that natural products make up at least some of the elements of more than 40 percent of all prescription drugs sold in the United States today is fundamental to the understanding of the importance of plants to health.

With virtually no health personnel and only home remedies, the means of preventing and treating illness were primitive prior to 1799. There have been radical changes in health care over the past two centuries. Medicine has grown from home remedies and folk cures into an effective discipline in the battle for assuring health.

Part I

Potluck Medicine
1799–1848

Dr. Saugrain gives notice of the first vaccine matter brought to St. Louis. Indigent persons, paupers, and Indians vaccinated gratuitously.

—May 1809 *Missouri Gazette* advertisement

Introduction

The greatest risk to health during the first half of the nineteenth century was the environment. Injuries from accidents or battles took a heavy toll, followed by fevers, the most common called "swamp fever." Diarrheas were common, though most were more often a nuisance than fatal. The existence and role of bacteria were unknown until the end of the century. Poor disposal of sewage fouled the water used for drinking, preparing food, and washing hands and utensils, leading to diarrhea, a disease called the flux, and cholera.

The population of the state grew rapidly after the Louisiana Purchase, with more than 75,000 people in St. Louis and 682,044 in the state by the mid-nineteenth century. Settlements sprang up along the Mississippi River. To the south of St. Louis, the Cape Girar-deau district had a population of 1,650, including 180 slaves, by 1804. In 1850 the population was 2,663.

Villages multiplied along the Missouri River with Boone's Lick in Howard County as the focal point. Benjamin Cooper led 70 men to the area in 1809. Legend says that Daniel Boone had hunted in Howard County and noted the high salt content of the spring. His sons, Nathan and Daniel Morgan Boone, had set up a salt plant as early as 1805. The spring water was boiled away in huge iron kettles, leaving the salt as residue. (Today, one of their kettles is displayed in the museum in the state capitol building in Jefferson City.) Pioneers used salt for curing meat and cooking, and the demand made the Boones' enterprise so successful that at one point they had as many as twenty workers. Boone's Lick grew from about 500 inhabitants to around 1,500 in 1821.

Pioneers traveling from Arkansas on the White River settled southwest Missouri around 1820. Springfield was the first settlement at the site, probably named after Springfield, Tennessee, the hometown of Kindred Rose, an early settler in the area. However Robert L. Ramsey favors another account of the naming of the town in 1833, as he reported in *Our Storehouse of Missouri Place Names:*

> The most authentic account tells us just how it was done: "Everybody in Greene County was invited to come in and vote their choice of a name for the county seat. James Wilson had a jug of white whiskey; and as fast as the people came in, he took them over to his tent and said: 'I am going to live here. I was born and raised in a beautiful little town in Massachusetts named Springfield; and it would please me very much if you would go over and vote to name this town *Springfield.*' Then he produced the jug . . ." Needless to say, Wilson had his way.

From 1837 to 1839, Cherokee groups passed near Springfield on their forced move from their home in the East to Indian Territory in present-day Oklahoma. Joan Gilbert in *The Trail of Tears across Missouri* tells of the hardship and sickness along the Cherokee route. Typhoid, measles, scarlet fever, flu, pneumonia, tuberculosis, and cholera afflicted great numbers, with cholera taking the greatest toll. The cold and lack of food caused misery and, often, deaths as the Cherokee crossed Missouri. One group, camped only two miles out of Springfield, buried four children and a woman before going on. Dr. W. I. I. Morrow, who traveled with the Richard Taylor detachment, ministered to the ill and injured but struggled without effective medicines.

Throughout Missouri, home remedies were all that stood between the afflicted and their deathbeds. The shaman or medicine man to the Indians and the preacher or missionary to the settlers dispensed such remedies. The birthing pains of the organized practice of medicine would be felt in a most inauspicious place, Arrow Rock.

1

Diseases and Injuries on the Trail

President Thomas Jefferson was interested in finding a water route from the Mississippi River to the Pacific Ocean, and even before the Louisiana Purchase, he authorized the Lewis and Clark Expedition, which left St. Charles in May 1804. Meriwether Lewis and William Clark led the expedition up the Missouri River to its source, then continued to the Pacific Ocean in search of a passage to the West Coast before returning to St. Louis in 1806. Their feat is especially remarkable in that with all the hardships they encountered and the threats by hostile Indians, only one person died, probably from a ruptured appendix. Clark not only led the company but also served as the group's doctor and treated such common ailments as fevers and diarrheas.

In 1806, three years after the U.S. purchased Louisiana for thirteen million dollars, territorial leaders in Upper Louisiana formed the first legislative body in what is now Missouri. It comprised one house with four members. Congress created the Missouri Territory six years later. At the time, they believed the name *Missouri* meant "muddy," a description taken from the muddy river. Researchers have since shown that the Indian meaning of Missouri was actually "people of large canoes."

In 1807, the territorial government sent a group to retrace the Lewis and Clark Expedition route. Their mission was to identify the several sources of the Missouri River. They were attacked by Blackfoot Indians 1,800 miles upriver from Arrow Rock. A young explorer, George Shannon, who had accompanied Lewis and Clark on the first trip up the Missouri River, was hit in the knee by a musket ball during the skirmish. He survived the long trip downriver to St. Louis, where Dr. Bernard Farrar, then in his early twenties, performed the first successful thigh amputation in Missouri. Years later when Shannon had become a famous judge, he said, "I owe my life and my honors to the Doctor."

In June 1808, road development began in Missouri. Two days after the Louisiana Territorial Legislature incorporated Ste. Genevieve as a town, it enacted a law to survey for a road from St. Louis to Ste. Genevieve to Cape Girardeau, which had just been established, and on to New Madrid. The old El Camino Real Trail was selected as the route to be followed. Within a few months, a supplement to the law directed that the road was to be twenty-five feet wide and built by volunteers. If workers did not step forward, judges in the districts along the route had the authority to order local men to work. By that time Ste. Genevieve was located three miles north of its original spot; the flood of 1785 had washed the first village away. By 1808 it had a population of 949, 24 more than St. Louis.

Two historical events struck the Missouri Territory early in the century, the New Madrid earthquakes of 1811–1812 and the war of 1812–1814 with England and her Indian allies. The earthquakes left more permanent scars on the land than did the war. With only 250 regular U.S. soldiers west of the Mississippi River, hostilities were limited to a series of skirmishes with the Indians, angry over loss of land, sickness brought by the white man, and other problems that had developed as the government of the territory changed hands.

The environment in Missouri changed as pioneers moved west and established farms and settlements. Travel along trails was dangerous and now posed the greatest risk to settlers' health. In 1813, the governor of the Missouri Territory, William Clark, sent George Sibley, who had been the Indian agent at Fort Osage, to build a blockhouse as a trading post in Arrow Rock. Cooper's Fort, located across the river, was not far from where the Boones processed salt. With these activities and the growth of Franklin, the area became the focal point for the development of trails for travel westward. Boone's Lick Road reached from St. Charles to Franklin and Arrow Rock. From there the Old Trails Road led to Fort Osage, twenty miles northwest of Boonville, on what is now

Highway 41 to Independence and Westport. The Santa Fe Trail headed southwest through Westport, Council Grove, and Fort Larned, to Santa Fe, New Mexico. Between Westport and Council Grove the trail split, and the northerly branch, the Oregon Trail, coursed along the Platte River to Fort Kearney, then to Fort Laramie, and on to Oregon.

Injuries, whether from accidents or from conflicts, often occurred and represented one health problem that was sometimes treatable. Thomas Hall in *Medicine on the Santa Fe Trail* writes about many injuries on the trail. In the book, Hall recounts one of the more serious accidents that occurred in 1826, as told to him in vivid detail by a Charles W. Gentry:

> Andrew Broaddus, a Missouri freighter formerly from Madison County, Kentucky, at his first sight of buffalo became excited and in attempting to draw his rifle, muzzle end first from his wagon, discharged its contents into his right arm . . . several days later at Walnut Creek gangrene had set in. The arm was bound tightly above the wound with a cord; the flesh was severed with a razor to the bone, which was quickly sawed off, and the flesh seared with a red hot coupling pin.

Travelers were also likely to contract diseases, probably from travel through swampy regions and exposure to crowds in congested stopping areas. Much as explorers had spread disease to the Indians, new people moving west brought illness to the residents of villages along the trails. Medicine had little help to offer for the common afflictions—measles, mumps, consumption and diphtheria, dysentery, smallpox, and typhoid. Scurvy, an ailment common to sailors and immigrants on long ocean voyages who were deprived of vitamin C, afflicted some.

Fortunately for those using the trails, Dr. John Sappington, the area's first physician, settled on a farm two miles west of Arrow Rock in 1819. He began dispensing his "anti-fever" medicine, quinine, as early as 1823 and practiced until 1832, when he quit to make and sell his famous medicine. He published the first medical book west of the Mississippi, a treatise on his medicine. In his book, *The Theory and Treatment of Fevers,* he hints at the controversy he faced when his theories were challenged, mostly by academicians in St. Louis and the East.

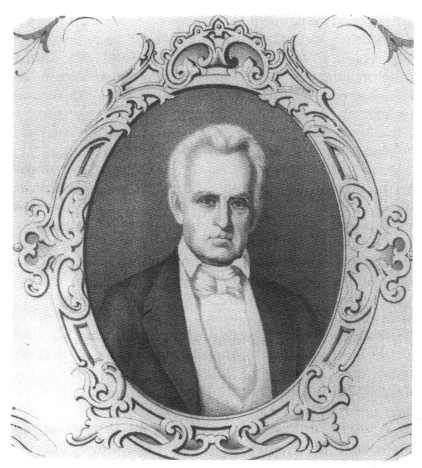

Dr. John Sappington recognized that quinine was the effective ingredient in the extract of Peruvian bark and sent his sons to Philadelphia to purchase large quantities of the bark. (State Historical Society of Missouri, Columbia)

In addition to medicine for malaria, smallpox vaccine was soon available to the traveler along the trails. Europe enjoyed the benefit of Dr. Edward Jenner's discovery of a vaccination to prevent smallpox in 1796, and Dr. Saugrain of St. Louis had the vaccine in his hands by 1809. While smallpox occurred less frequently than many other afflictions, it was frightening because it often caused death or disfigurement. Sappington's medicine and smallpox vaccine protected the people who accompanied Meredith M. Marmaduke and Augustus Storrs on their successful trip to Santa Fe in 1824. President John Quincy Adams appointed Maj. George Sibley the following year as one of three commissioners to "lay out a road from Fort Osage to Mexico," for the Santa Fe Trail. Sappington's "anti-fever" medicine protected the road workers as well as Sibley during his negotiations with Indian tribes occupying the lands along the trail.

Meredith Marmaduke, who married one of Sappington's daughters in 1826, made six trips in all to Santa Fe. He became Missouri's eighth governor when Thomas Reynolds committed suicide eight months before the end of his term, but he did not receive his party's nomination for a full term. He went back to Arrow Rock and is buried in the same cemetery as Sappington, along with another Missouri governor, Claiborne Fox Jackson.

In spite of his medical skill, Dr. Sappington could not protect his family from frontier conditions. For example, Claiborne Fox Jackson married one of Sappington's daughters, Jane. When she died six months after the wedding, he married a second daughter, Louisa. After she was killed in an accident, he asked for the hand of Sappington's oldest daughter, Eliza. According to John Hert of Fayette, legend has it that the crusty old doctor gave his consent but growled, "Well, you can have her, son, but if you come back for the old lady [the doctor's wife] I'll have to say no."

Although many physicians scoffed at Sappington's medicine, and the St. Louis Medical Society, which was incorporated in 1837 as the Medical Society of Missouri, denied him membership, he continued to promote its use so successfully that he invited Dr. George Penn to join his practice in 1832 as a junior partner to help him tend patients. Dr. Penn was ambitious and became renowned in his own right. He traveled the Santa Fe Trail as chief surgeon in Col. Alexander Doniphan's regiment in 1846. He also played an important role in the formation of the Missouri Medical Society in 1853, though he declined the offer to serve as the society's president, perhaps in deference to Dr. Sappington.

A favorite stopping place for people on the trails as well as on the river, Arrow Rock grew rapidly. Joseph Huston, a pioneer en-

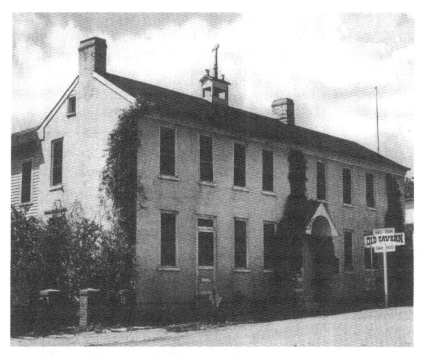

Arrow Rock Tavern was built by John Huston for travelers along the Boone's Lick Trail and the Missouri River. For twenty-five cents a traveler could sleep in the upstairs bedroom, where two small beds frequently held three travelers each. A few more people could bed down on blankets on the floor. A meal and a bath from a washbowl were included in the price, making it a real bargain. (State Historical Society of Missouri, Columbia)

trepreneur, built Arrow Rock Tavern in 1834 to house travelers. Huston served as county judge, justice of the peace, and later, village postmaster. He ran a store and tavern and dispensed a variety of home medicines.

The movement of goods and people by boat soon added to the flow of westward migration. It was faster and easier to move great quantities of goods over the water, and the numbers of pioneers traveling upriver grew rapidly. The *Independence* was the first steamboat to ascend the Missouri, arriving in Franklin, the "Queen

City" of the Boone's Lick towns, in May 1819. The *Missouri Intelligencer,* in business again after a three-year lapse, captured the excitement of the citizens in its September 27 publication:

ARRIVAL of the STEAM BOAT INDEPENDENCE

... the 28th [May] ult. the citizens of Franklin, with the most lively emotions of pleasure, witnessed the arrival of this beautiful boat, owned and commanded by Captain Nelson, of Louisville. Her approach to the landing was greeted by a federal salute, accompanied with the acclamations of an admiring crowd, who had assembled on the bank of the river for the purpose of viewing this novel and interesting sight.

In 1821, Pierre Laclede and Francois Chouteau established a trading post at what is now Kansas City. The *Independence* inaugurated riverboat traffic and the settlement of towns along the river as far as St. Joseph, where Joseph Robidoux had established a trading post in the mid–1820s.

Along with the advantages of river travel came added risks to health, greater than with travel by land for two reasons: a single accident could result in large numbers of injured and dead, and the spread of disease was more rapid as passengers and crew mingled with settlers along the river. The ever-changing course of the Missouri River and the snags, logs, and sandbars were responsible for a large number of steamboat accidents. In 1853, the explosion of the *Saluda* at Lexington killed 100 Mormons. That year 466 people were killed in 67 steamboat accidents.

In 1817 the territorial legislature had petitioned Congress for statehood. The process quickly became embroiled in the "slave versus free state" battle, which Congress finally resolved by coupling Missouri's petition for statehood with that of Maine. President Madison proclaimed Missouri's admission into the Union in August 1821, and the state was born. In 1826 the General Assembly of Missouri moved the state capital by flatboat from its temporary home in St. Charles to Jefferson City, and settlement along the river continued to increase. Northerly growth along the Mississippi also was significant as towns became locations for

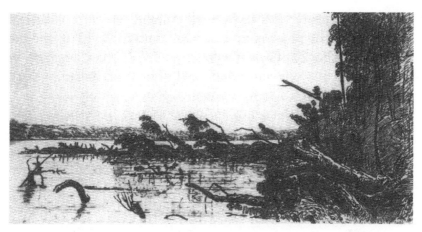

The Missouri River in the early 1800s was dangerous for steamboats. Snags and the continuous changes in the course of the main channel caused numerous accidents. By 1850, 441 vessels had sunk or been damaged in the Missouri River with a great loss of life and goods. (State Historical Society of Missouri, Columbia)

loading barges. Above the Mississippi River floodplain Hawkins Smith built the first gristmill on the South River near Palmyra in 1818. The town of Hannibal began in 1819 with lots at the mouth of the Bear River on the Mississippi awarded to Abraham Bird as compensation for New Madrid earthquake losses. Samuel Stone began a ferry service across the Mississippi River in 1831, and by 1840, the population had grown to 1,034. Among the residents was five-year-old Samuel Clemens, who would later call himself Mark Twain.

The incorporation of St. Joseph in 1845, directly across the state from Hannibal, played an important role in the next step in transportation. In February 1847 the general assembly incorporated the Hannibal–St. Joseph Railroad, the first to cross the state and the only state-aided railroad never to default. The last spike would be driven near Chillicothe in February 1859.

Many other exciting developments accompanied the establishment of roads, the increase in steamboat travel, and the development of firm plans for a cross-state railroad. The first theatrical performance took place in St. Louis on January 14, 1814, and the first public school in the city opened in 1838. The University of Missouri, the first state university west of the Mississippi, opened in April 1841 with sixty-two students listed.

The exciting achievements in transportation, governance, culture, and education during these fifty years brought a rapid growth in population that strained crowded, poorly planned cities. Progress in medicine could not keep pace with the health problems spawned by these changes; however, the use of quinine and the smallpox vaccine, two major medical innovations before 1849, offset somewhat the absence of standards and regulations in community health and medical education.

2

Growth of Education and Number of Physicians

By the early 1800s, the latest medical advances in Europe had reached the larger American cities, including St. Louis. New doctors soon arrived to join the handful of physicians practicing in St. Louis at the turn of the century. Dr. Antoine Francois Saugrain arrived in St. Louis from Gallipolis, Ohio. Born in Paris in 1763, the thirty-seven-year-old physician was highly educated, grounded in chemistry, mineralogy, and use of drugs. In the 1780s the king of Spain had sent Saugrain to Mexico to explore mines there. In 1790 he made his third trip to America, joining a number of French families who had decided to settle on land offered by the Scioto Company in Gallipolis, Ohio, after the French Revolution. The Ohio settlement struggled, prompting Saugrain to move to St. Louis in 1804. There he made sulfur matches for the Lewis and Clark Expedition while he established a medical practice. Appointed "Jefferson Surgeon" of the U.S. Army at Fort Belle Fontaine in 1805, Saugrain became the senior surgical officer at the fort.

Letters from his mother in Paris, now held in the Missouri Historical Society in St. Louis, speak of the terrors of the Revolution, the reign of Napoleon Bonaparte, her reduced income, and inoculations being introduced by an English doctor. In 1801 she wrote that she feared to write again because of the risk that his name would be placed on the list of "émigrés." Napoleon had persuaded Spain to cede the Louisiana Territory back to France in 1800, and for a time, he dreamed of establishing a French empire in the western hemisphere. His hand extended to the New World, where French emigrants were listed as enemies. Those who were captured were imprisoned or executed.

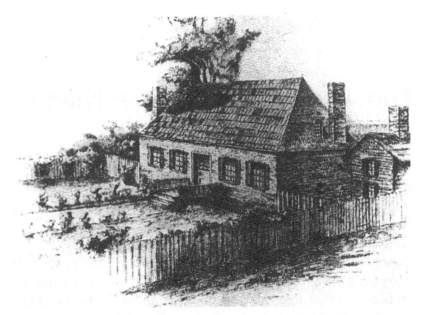

Dr. Antoine Saugrain's residence and garden in St. Louis. Throughout his years as an army surgeon, Dr. Saugrain continued to practice in St. Louis until his death in 1820. He gained a great reputation for the introduction of smallpox vaccine in 1809 and for his considerable charitable work. (Missouri Historical Society, St. Louis)

Known as the father of the medical profession in St. Louis, Dr. Bernard G. Farrar, the first American-born physician to move to Missouri, was the next to arrive in St. Louis. In 1810, Dr. Farrar became known from his involvement in a duel over a card game. Both he and his opponent—James Graham—were wounded, and Graham eventually died from his wounds. Farrar served St. Louis during the War of 1812 and gained fame from one of his stranger cases. E. J. Goodwin, M.D., in *A History of Medicine in Missouri,* gives the following account of an event that contributed to Farrar's reputation as a physician:

> The Doctor was summoned to see a female who had been sick for some time and was considered to be dead by her friends and the physicians. Indeed her shroud was being made and the corpse had been laid

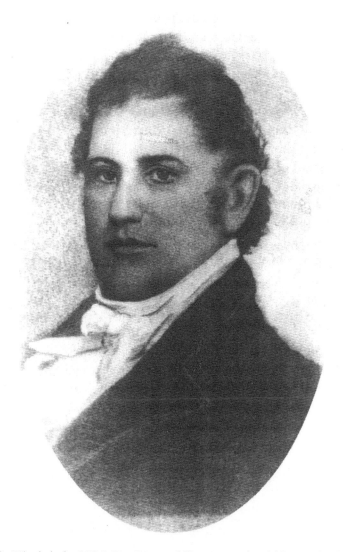

Born in Virginia in 1785, Dr. Bernard Farrar received his medical training at Transylvania University in Kentucky and moved to St. Louis in 1806. Within a year of his arrival he showed his courage and abilities by performing the amputation on George Shannon. (State Historical Society of Missouri, Columbia)

out when the Doctor appeared. The mirror and other usual tests of vitality were applied but with negative results. The idea now struck the doctor to apply a red hot smoothing iron to the soles of her feet. This was soon done, whereupon the woman stood erect and cried aloud. She returned to perfect health.

Dr. Farrar's practice flourished until the cholera epidemic of 1849. Exhausted from months of treating hundreds of afflicted patients, he contracted cholera himself and died. He was sixty-four.

The spread of physicians throughout the state was rapid. A Dr. John Brown opened an office in Jefferson City in 1819, although Dr. Joseph Summers's book *Medical Milestones in Cole County, Missouri* (1998) expresses doubts about his qualifications: "Although Dr. Brown claimed to be a physician, his credentials are questionable." In the early 1820s, Stephen Doriss started private practice in the area. By 1840 eighteen physicians had arrived in Cole County.

Dr. Lowry of Franklin announced in the *Missouri Intelligencer* on April 23, 1819, that he was "Thankful for the encouragement received in his services to the citizens of Howard and Cooper Counties, in the practice of Medicine, Surgery, and Midwifery and hopes to merit patronage." Clay County in western Missouri, established in 1822, finally enjoyed the services of a physician in 1832 when Dr. Joseph Wood moved from Kentucky. Early on, Dr. Wood used quinine for swamp fever.

Pettis County boasted three physicians. Dr. Christian Bidstrap came from Denmark to settle in Georgetown in 1833. That same year Dr. Moses Ferris arrived in Longwood. They practiced for eight and ten years, respectively. In 1834 Dr. William Westfield began practice in Georgetown.

Perhaps the most famous physician at that time was Dr. William Beaumont. In 1834 the army transferred Beaumont to the Jefferson Barracks, located fourteen miles south of St. Louis. The previous year he had published results of his research carried out on Alexis St. Martin, a Canadian of French descent, injured in an accident at a trading post on an island where the waters of Lake Michigan and Lake Huron join. Recognized today as the most sig-

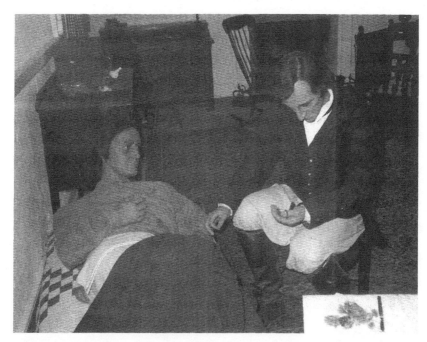

The officers' stone quarters building, built in 1780 inside the walls of Fort Mackinac, has been restored to show the personal quarters of Dr. William Beaumont. When the town commission stopped financial support for the prolonged recovery of Alexis St. Martin, Dr. Beaumont took his prize patient into his home and, as shown by these lifelike figures, studied the digestive processes of the stomach through the wound in St. Martin's side. The quarters consisted of a small bedroom for Dr. Beaumont, his wife of two years, and one-year-old daughter and this room, where St. Martin slept and where the family ate, played, and carried out social activities. Deborah Green Platt, a Quaker widow when Beaumont married her, supported her husband's kind actions toward St. Martin. Beaumont, however, was not simply being kind. He was also taking advantage of an opportunity to carry out research on a subject never before investigated.

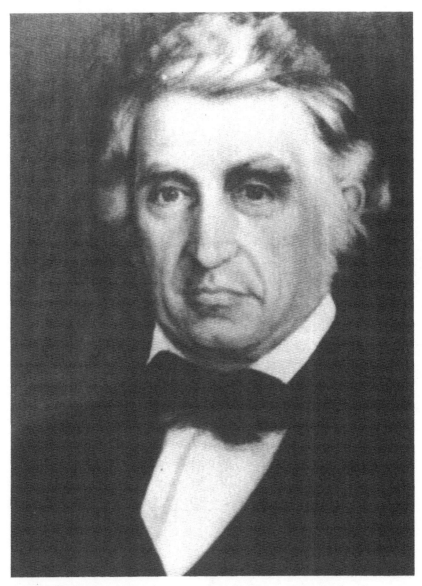

Dr. William Beaumont served as vice president of the St. Louis Medical Society in 1838. Burdened with a busy practice, he resigned from the army in 1840. (State Historical Society of Missouri, Columbia)

nificant clinical research of its day, the studies by Beaumont described physiology of the stomach from experiments conducted on St. Martin, who had survived a gunshot wound to the abdomen. The wound was not lethal although it made a hole in the victim's stomach. Luckily, stomach juices and food drained through the bullet tract to the outside instead of into the abdominal cavity, which would have led to peritonitis and death. This rare circumstance and the skill of Beaumont (the surgeon at nearby Fort Mackinac) in treating the wound, saved St. Martin's life. Recovery was so difficult Beaumont took St. Martin into his own home and continued treating him over three years. When Beaumont transferred to the St. Louis Arsenal as its medical officer, however, he could not convince St. Martin to join him.

In 1835, Beaumont started medical practice in the city, and in 1843, Mary Dugan, a patient who developed drainage after he did a hernia repair, sued him. According to Reginald Horsman in *Frontier Doctor,* Dugan sued Beaumont for ten thousand dollars, claiming the drainage through the incision was from an injury to the intestine that had occurred during his operation. Some experts thought she was correct, but others thought she had tuberculosis of the intestine, a fairly common form of tuberculosis at the time, caused by unpasteurized milk. In 1848 a jury acquitted Beaumont, and he continued his successful surgical practice in St. Louis until his death in 1853. He died following a fall down the steps of a patient's home.

Across the state, Dr. Leo Twyman practiced in Westport for one year and then moved to Independence in 1845 and set up practice. In 1847, the brother of Gov. Lilburn Boggs, Dr. Joseph Boggs, joined his medical practice. The first physician in Kansas City was Dr. Benoist Troost. Born in Holland and educated in Paris, he settled in Missouri in 1845. In 1848 Isaac M. Ridge, born in 1825 and educated at Transylvania University in Kentucky, arrived.

St. Joseph, the Buchanan County seat and the largest city in western Missouri, served as the main departure point for emigrants. In the years 1849 and 1850, over 100,000 people passed through on their way west. Its importance as a gateway to the West accounts for its having eleven physicians for fewer than 1,500 residents.

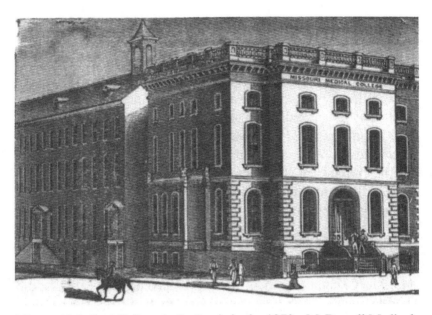

Missouri Medical College in St. Louis in the 1870s. McDowell Medical College, named after Dr. Joseph McDowell, professor of anatomy, had started as a medical department of Kemper College, which opened in 1838 in St. Louis. (State Historical Society of Missouri, Columbia)

As midcentury approached, pharmacies and a few hospitals offered help in treating diseases and dispensing remedies most common during this period. Most physicians, all educated outside of Missouri, set up practices in the more populated counties, although a few others scattered across the state. The need for physicians, which grew along with the state's population and the increase in injuries and diseases, led to establishment of medical training in the state in the 1840s. Although a young state, Missouri had demonstrated its interest in higher education in 1832, when the legislature granted a charter for the formation of St. Louis University. This interest set the stage for medical education. At the urging of St. Louis physicians, the university formed a medical department, which opened to students in 1841. Dr. Charles A. Pope came to St. Louis in 1842 as dean of the department and professor of anatomy.

In 1847 John Hiram Lathrop, president of the University of Missouri, endorsed an affiliation between McDowell Medical College and the University of Missouri to form a medical department in St. Louis to be called Missouri Medical College.

The City Hospital of St. Louis, measuring 111 by 50 feet and costing $17,000, opened in June 1846. Built for 90 patients, it served St. Louis until 1856 when fire destroyed it. The cost to rebuild it in 1857 was $62,000.

Dispersion of physicians throughout the state, establishment of pharmacies, and construction of hospitals served as visual proof to the public of advances in medicine. But had the diagnosis of disease improved? And could physicians cure ailments?

3

Home Remedies, Smallpox Vaccine, and Quinine

From Saugrain's announcement in the newspaper, we know small-pox vaccination was available in St. Louis early in the century. Its use by those passing through Arrow Rock on their way to Santa Fe and Oregon proves it had spread out of St. Louis into central Missouri. Thomas Hall in *Medicine on the Santa Fe Trail* noted that the Pawnee, traditional enemies of the Osage, lost half their people to a terrible epidemic of smallpox in 1831. Dr. Victor Trexier, the French physician who spent part of the 1840s with the Osage, remarked that the freedom of pockmarks among the Osage was due to their having received smallpox vaccinations some years previously.

Arrow Rock was the site of other medical progress. Use of quinine, except by an occasional physician around the state, was restricted to the Boone's Lick area. The medical establishment continued to ridicule Sappington, and the professors at the university medical school in St. Louis made strong efforts to discredit his use of quinine for swamp fever. Marmaduke's and Doniphan's forces believed in quinine, as they had seen its benefit in their travels. But most doctors used calomel, a traditional purgative long used to clean out the intestines. Medical schools taught that this cleansing would rid the body of bad humors causing fever, diarrhea, and about any disease except diabetes. For diabetes and other mysterious ailments they removed from a half-pint to a pint of blood.

Dr. Daniel Johnson of Palmyra wrote in the February 1840 *Palmyra Missouri Whig and General Advisor:*

> I own that calomel practice is both cheap and easy to the physician,
> for the whole extent of both theory and practice is, to give calomel, if

that will not help, double and treble the dose of calomel. If the patient recovers, calomel cured him . . . if he dies, nothing in the world would have saved him.

This attitude cost many Missourians their lives. An editorial in the September–October 1871 issue of the *Kansas City Medical Journal* stated: "The slow recognition of quinine resulted in more deaths than the late [Civil] war."

Without quinine for swamp fever or vaccination for smallpox, the physician had no medicine for their cure. For all other ailments, treatments would occasionally make the patient feel better but would never cure him. Some medicines were so harsh they made the patient's condition worse.

In Lanser's *Pioneer Physician,* Dr. Johnson of Palmyra said: "The physician who guessed correctly more frequently than his colleagues was the best doctor." No instruments or blood tests existed. Doctors had only their eyes and hands to make diagnoses.

Compared with treatment of diseases, the care of penetrating wounds had advanced somewhat. In the days of the Napoleonic wars, doctors poured boiling oil into a wound. During the War of 1812 with the British, in which attacks were mainly by Indians, doctors treated gunshot or arrow wounds by first attempting to extract the bullet or arrowhead and then burning the wound with a red-hot object. This had some merit in principle; its purpose was to remove the foreign object, as well as any bits of clothing it had carried with it into the flesh. But because doctors did not yet know what caused infection, they made no attempt to keep bacteria out of the wound. Some bacteria probably got carried into the wound by the arrow, knife, or bullet, but dirty hands and instruments introduced much more. Because wounds involving a body cavity— the head, chest, or abdomen—were generally fatal, no attempt was made to remove the missile. Pressure or a tourniquet usually succeeded in stopping the bleeding. But if the wound was probed, infection occurred, frequently causing death.

A few individuals, those with wounds that were near the surface, small, or drained well, survived such primitive techniques. Deadly infection could quickly spread through the person's entire

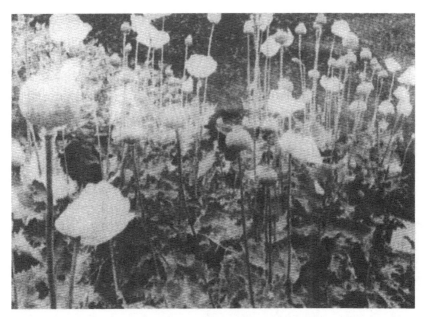

Poppy fields in Lucknow, India, where one acre yields twenty-five to thirty-five kilograms of opium, depending on several factors, such as type of soil, time of sowing, weather conditions, and the number of lancings. Two to three weeks after the petals fall, the capsule of the plant is lanced to obtain the medicinal chemicals, the more important ones being codeine, papaverine, and morphine. (Haworth Press, June 16, 1999)

system. For someone with a severe wound in the arm or leg, doctors usually had to amputate to prevent the infection from spreading or because the limb had become gangrenous from interrupted blood flow below the wound. Since there were no drugs to fight infection, doctors usually amputated right away. They did not wait for signs of infection to appear for most moderate to severe wounds, especially of the penetrating type, reasoning that, by acting immediately, they would prevent spread of infection into the bloodstream and save life. Unfortunately, they did not wash their hands or use antiseptics. And what was worse, they reused dirty, bloody instruments, practically guaranteeing that the amputation stump would become infected, leading to blood poisoning, and kill the patient.

Physicians had opium in various forms for pains associated with disease, but no anesthesia. The surgeon gave the patient whiskey or had him "bite the bullet." Although Crawford Long, a physician in Georgia, had used ether for anesthesia to remove skin tumors in 1842, and William Morton, a dentist in Massachusetts, had used ether in a hospital operating room in 1846, this method of pain relief for operations was not available to Missouri physicians until much later. Without anesthesia, antibiotics, or blood for transfusion, physicians of the time did not attempt operations on wounds of the body cavities.

Missourians treated all but the most severe injuries with home remedies. By 1833 several medical books written for the general public were available and in many Missouri homes. They were not just used in remote areas. Even in cities, the tools available to physicians for rendering a diagnosis and the drugs to treat illness were so few that it is not surprising that people tried home remedies first.

Goiter was common and easily recognized. In *The American Gentleman's Medical Pocket-Book and Health Adviser,* published in 1833, James Kay wrote that the causes of goiter were "supposed to consist of some peculiarities in the water where they occur." After making that astute observation for the time, Kay stated it was not treatable. By the end of the nineteenth century, physicians knew that goiters were common in the Midwest because of insufficient iodine in the water and that using iodized salt would prevent them. Removal of goiters became a common operation.

Kay's book gave general directions for care of accident victims: "Whenever a blow has been inflicted, whether by being thrown from a horse, out of a carriage, by falling from a height, or any other way, bleed the patient to the amount of 12 or 14 ounces on the spot if practicable, if not, as soon as possible."

Asthma, a condition physicians thought occurred rarely before puberty, had its seat in the "pneumo-gastric nerve," a nonexistent nerve invented by the medical "experts." In July 1834, the Jefferson City paper suggested a home remedy of "the best mocha newly burned, with or without milk or sugar."

Physicians had diagnosed cholera by the middle of this period. Robyn Burnett and Ken Luebbering in *German Settlement in Missouri: New Land, Old Ways* note that German immigrants frequently died of cholera on their way to America or died after arrival. Frederick Steines and his family arrived in St. Louis in the summer of 1834. Among the city's seven thousand residents were about eighteen German families and a few unmarried Germans. By the end of July, Steines's wife and four children had died of cholera. The immigrants also suffered from other ailments. Burnett and Luebbering have documented some of the health problems of the German immigrants. For example, Dr. Bernhard Bruns and his twenty-three–year-old wife moved to Westphalia in 1836. Three of their four children died of dysentery in 1841. Typhoid brought death as well, taking the life of Paul Follenius, brother-in-law of Friedrich Muench, in 1844. The two men, noted for their plans to concentrate German immigrants in a territory in the West to establish a German state in the Union, had settled in Warren County in 1834.

Knowledge of diseases gradually increased however. By the nineteenth century doctors recognized many common ailments, although they did not understand their causes. In the absence of scientific methods, physicians were forced to guess at the causes of diseases. For example, diabetes had been recognized in ancient Rome, but when the medical experts of the nineteenth century pointed out the lack of understanding of the Romans, they showed their own misconceptions about diseases. In *Practice of Medicine,* published in 1835, John Eberle, M.D., professor of materia medica and botany in the Ohio Medical College, commented on the poor understanding of diabetes held by the ancients: "It does not appear that they had any knowledge of the essential characteristic of the disease, namely, the saccharin characteristic of the disease." Experts of Eberle's time held several incorrect theories on the nature of the diabetes. Some claimed it was due to a laxity of the kidneys, and many pathologists thought the "primary seat of diabetes [to be] in the liver." The treatment was venesection, local bleeding by leeches and cups, "with excellent effect."

Whooping cough was common in adults and children, but its

cause was a mystery. Dr. Eberle said, "There exists no other cause, so far as we know, capable of producing this affliction, than the peculiar contagion which is generated by the disease itself. . . . cold in conjunction with humidity may give rise . . . all these diseases such as measles arise from accidental causes."

The years 1799 to 1848 were hard but exciting for settlers in Missouri; the territory became a state, and areas in all parts of the state drew immigrants both from the eastern United States and from the impoverished countries of Europe. By the early 1820s, according to Charles van Ravenswaay, St. Louis had become a

> pageant of nationalities, each with its own characteristic dress. In addition to the native-born Americans and Creoles, St. Louis had Italians, Poles, Germans, Swiss, Jews, French, English, Irish, Dutch, Indians, and Africans. . . . Old world costumes mixed with outfits typical of the American West. Priests and nuns in black were somber foils for the army officers in their colorful uniforms. Aristocratic Creole women dressed in the latest Parisian fashion.

Jesse Benton, the daughter of Senator Thomas Hart Benton, attended a French school when her family was in St. Louis, and in her remembrances written many years later, she gave vivid descriptions of the city during the early years of statehood, when a mingling of cultures and languages brought color and excitement, and cholera brought fear and death. Born in 1824, she witnessed the cholera epidemic of 1832.

> So in the summer I was about eight, this bright careless St. Louis life seemed to chill over. At first we were only told we were not to go to school. Then, we were to play only with each other in our own grounds and no more little friends visited us or we them. The friends who came to my father on the long gallery were . . . quick and busy in coming and going, and all looked grave. . . . We saw many, many funerals passing. . . soon drays with many coffins piled on jolted fast along the rough street.
>
> All the water was brought in large barrels from the river and poured, bucket by bucket, into great jars of red earthenware, some of them five feet high. These jars had their own large cool room paved with glazed red brick and level with the street. The jars of drinking water and for

cooking were clarified of the mud of the river by alum and blanched almonds. So much was needed now that even we children were useful in this sort of work. In that cool dark room the melons used to be kept, but there were no melons or fruit now—we ate only rice and mutton and such simple things.

Jesse's mother fell ill of cholera, just as "all seemed safe," but recovered. "It was a bad illness, but with that one brush of the dark angel's wing our house stood as before."

The cholera and other diseases were to return throughout the nineteenth century, but progress continued. The roads were still dirt trails with deeply worn ruts in some places that turned to quagmires with rain, but aided by riverboats, the rapid movement of people and goods increased. Local and state governments came into being, enacting legislation, at least near the end of the period, that was of little benefit before 1850 but would begin benefiting communities during the next half century.

Part II
Community Medicine
1849–1898

In a real sense the war between the states brought forth a medical revolution and, perhaps above all, an awareness of public health.
—Stewart Brooks, *Civil War Medicine,* 1966

Introduction

In the mid–1800s, Missouri saw changes that were to affect the lives of all its citizens. Railroads made it possible to build cities away from the Missouri River, but the means for more rapid distribution of goods also allowed more rapid spread of disease. The Civil War created lasting social tensions between Missouri and neighboring states and among groups within the state. The meager medical lessons learned from the war hardly compensated for the tragic losses of life and the economic scars that resulted.

The developments of the previous fifty years had set the stage for some advances in medicine. Increased numbers of villages and towns, riverboats, and many untrained physicians now forced Missourians to catch up to the rest of the country. Demand for statewide movement of goods and people, plus overcrowding in poorly planned (or completely unplanned) cities forced the newly elected legislators to begin establishing methods to provide statewide transportation. Contagious diseases, which already traveled easily, were disseminated more rapidly, compelling officials to try to regulate matters that affected health, including the training of physicians. Over the next fifty years regulation and organization replaced expansion. One important development was the organization in 1853 of the Missouri Medical Society, replacing the St. Louis Medical Society. Originally incorporated in 1837 as the Medical Society of Missouri, the organization had been inactive for a decade. The reorganized society quickly embarked on a campaign to set standards for medical ethics, an effort in which Dr. George Penn, Dr. Sappington's former partner, took an active part.

4

Evils of Cities and Medical School Problems

Several tragic events that were to have lasting consequences occurred at midcentury. In 1849 a fire devastated a large part of St.
Louis. It started when the steamer *White Cloud,* a small three
thousand–dollar boat, caught fire. The blaze jumped to nearby
boats and to tons of cargo on the levee and then spread to down-
town St. Louis, where it destroyed fifteen blocks of businesses and
houses.

The cholera epidemic of 1849 may have begun as early as
November 1848. A sudden increase in the number of cases of diarrhea appeared that month, but the rapid rise in deaths common to
cholera did not follow immediately.

The disease broke out in New Orleans in December 1848, and
several steamboats carried infected passengers to St. Louis.
Physicians diagnosed the first case in St. Louis on January 5,
1849, in a stout, healthy laboring man. He died the following day.
They reported the next, an Irish boatman, on January 7, and the
third on the seventeenth. The deaths mounted; 33 had died by the
end of January. When the year ended, officials had recorded 8,603
deaths from all causes for St. Louis, a town of 70,000. Of these,
records showed that cholera caused 4,557 deaths, 2,173 in children five years of age and under. The steamboat *Timour* carried
cholera to Jefferson City later in 1849. It broke out in the village
of Westphalia that summer, taking the lives of one-third of the
population. Deaths persisted, though at a much slower rate, in sub-
sequent years. In July 1852, German immigrant Franz von Dawen
arrived in St. Louis with a slight touch of diarrhea. By the next day
he had developed a severe case of cholera, and he died before
seven that evening. His brother Adam wrote to the family in

Germany of the epidemics that had struck St. Louis again and again: "Cholera has made its appearance every summer since 1849 and has snatched away thousands of inhabitants of St. Louis. . . . This terrible disease has caused countless wounds which will not be healed soon." Workers laying the railroad took the disease to Hermann in 1854. Deaths from cholera averaged about eight hundred a year until 1866 when another epidemic hit St. Louis, this time brought in by rail. That year 3,527 people died from cholera. In 1873, 392 inhabitants of St. Louis died from the disease.

The sporadic appearance of cholera earlier in the century had gained the attention of health officials and even the legislature, which had expressed its interest in improving waste and water systems. The epidemic of 1849 forced the legislature to back laws with money; they allocated funds for improved sewage systems and drainage of polluted water from lakes and ponds.

Developments in means of travel and communication sometimes overshadowed the tragedies of epidemics. Railroads received a jump start in December 1850 when Gov. Austin A. King recommended that the state allocate money to support the development of several railroad lines. By 1859 the legislature had authorized twenty-four million dollars in state bonds for seven Missouri railroads. Although all but the Hannibal–St. Joseph Railroad defaulted on the bonds, the railroads soon passed riverboats as the main means of moving goods and people.

Jackson County incorporated the "Town Kansas City" in 1850. Trapper Daniel Morgan Boone had frequented the site in the 1790s. A permanent settlement began in 1821 when Francois Chouteau, with thirty pirogues and canoes, established the American Fur Company trading post near the junction of the Kaw and Missouri Rivers. Louis Grand Louis and Jacques Fannais settled there in 1825. Between 1860 and 1865 the population dropped from 7,180 to 3,500, but after the Civil War the area began to grow again. By 1870 the inhabitants numbered 32,260, compared with the 310,864 in St. Louis at that time.

Rapid communication came to Missouri when telegraph workers strung lines from St. Louis to Jefferson City in 1850 and from St. Louis to St. Joseph in 1850–1851. For points west, man and horse replaced the telegraph; in April 1860 the first Pony Express rider took the buckskin mail pouch and rode the ferry across the Missouri River at St. Joseph to begin the first leg of the 1,980–mile trip to Sacramento.

The Civil War had a devasting social and economic impact on Missouri. Less serious was the effect on the environment, although some battlefields blighted the landscape. The border war with Kansas had scarred western Missouri, and Union troops burned the town of Nevada in May 1863 to retaliate for the killing of six Federal militiamen by bushwhackers. The Bushwhacker Museum in Nevada has preserved records of the unsavory events of that time. The jail, which escaped the Union torch because it rested on the property of Thomas Austin, who had "decently taken care of the remains" of the bushwhacked Federal soldiers, stands behind the museum. Throughout the state neighbor fought neighbor and even brothers were on opposing sides. Many who fought with the Confederates, as well as others who were labeled Southern sympathizers, lost businesses, farms, and homes.

St. Louis seemed to be the crucial center for wounded in the war. In August 1, 1861, the U.S. government opened the New House of Refuge Hospital two miles south of the city. Hospital boats brought wounded from Illinois and other points east, and trains arrived from other locations with the wounded and sick. At the Battle of Wilson's Creek, a few miles southwest of Springfield, a bullet from Dockery's Fifth Arkansas Infantry hit Gen. Nathaniel Lyon in the heart. Friedrich Muench's youngest son, a Union soldier, also died in that battle. He was seventeen. The Union lost 300 men, and 700 more were wounded; 1,500 Confederates died, and from 2,000 to 2,500 were wounded.

Rev. Robert A. Austin was a chaplain in Gen. William Slack's Southern Division. In 1932 his grandson, Dr. C. S. Austin of Carrollton, published the account Austin wrote of his experience in the *Missouri Historical Review*. Austin remembered the stench of the battlefield from his work as a nurse in the field hospital: "A truce was called so we could retrieve the wounded from the battlefield. Many of the Confederate wounded were taken in wagons with the wounded Union soldiers to hospitals in Springfield."

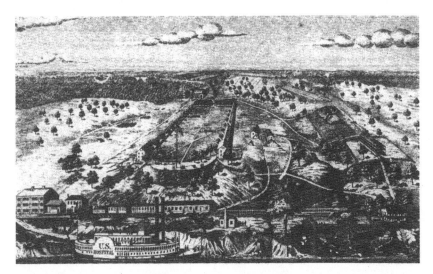

Hospital in St. Louis with hospital ship in the foreground and train with converted ambulance cars behind it. Apparently Robert Austin was not aware that 721 of the Confederate and Union soldiers wounded in the Battle of Wilson's Creek were ultimately transported to St. Louis by railcar. (Missouri Nurses Association, Jefferson City, courtesy State Historical Society of Missouri, Columbia)

Wagons converted into ambulances carried the more severely wounded to Pilot Knob, where ambulance cars of the Ironton Railroad carried them to the New House of Refuge Hospital in St. Louis. Due to the large number of wounded that poured into St. Louis, a shortage of food, medicine, clothing, buildings, and trained nurses caused such misery and so many deaths that the citizens of the city formed the Western Sanitary Commission to raise private funds to support care for the wounded. General Fremont gave his approval for the commission in September 1861. He appointed Dorothea Lynde Dix, a prominent social worker in St. Louis, as the general supervisor of female nurses in the military hospitals. Dix had distinguished herself the previous decade in Kansas by pushing for social change against many practices that imposed harsh restrictions on women in that state. Her appointment played an important role in the development of nursing in Missouri. Prior to the War between the States, religious orders had carried out nursing duties throughout the United States. Early in the war, recuperating soldiers also served as nurses.

Dix had strict standards for applicants. She considered only single women over the age of thirty, plain, dressed in brown or black, with no bows, curls, or jewelry, and no hoop skirts. Neither religious tenets nor inconsiderate physicians could stand between Dix's nurses and patient care. The women took on a fundamental role that would grow in significance as science began to revolutionize medicine. Nursing had staked its claim as the protector of the patient, offering comfort and honoring his wishes.

In 1862, three more hospitals opened in St. Louis, the Marine Hospital, Jefferson Barracks, and the Lawson. By March 1864 they had treated 11,434 patients, so that by the winter of 1864–1865, St. Louis had become a key area for sick war prisoners, with 818 in hospitals. That year 50 percent of those in the hospital would die.

The Civil War extracted a price from a large number of Missourians who fought outside the state. The Missouri Eighteenth headed North after completing Sherman's march through Georgia. John A. Drake of Hatfield's B Company was typical of the casualties of the war. According to an account in *The Eighteenth Missouri* by Leslie Anders, Drake had joined the unit at Laclede in November 1861 and after all the encounters in Sherman's march to the sea, died in Virginia. The Eighteenth had marched across battlefields between Richmond and the Potomac. "The sergeant was felled by sunstroke at Hanover Courthouse. Doctor Randolph worked over him all night but he died in the morning."

Statistics from the Eighteenth show that of those who joined, one-third were wounded, captured, or killed. Of those who died, 77 were killed in battle, 8 in mishaps, and 192 contracted a fatal disease. Wounds were not always fatal; 104 of the surviving soldiers were wounded, and some of them were part of the 198 in Confederate prisons. One hundred three soldiers deserted, and 198 were discharged for disabilities.

Table 1 lists the infectious diseases that struck the Federal army compared to the Confederate forces from May 1861 to December 31, 1862, and their associated mortality rates.

Table 1. *Comparison of Diseases between Confederate and Federal Forces* *

	Confederate		Federal	
Disease	**# cases**	**# deaths**	**# cases**	**# deaths**
Typhus/typhoid fever	36,746	12,225	51,571	11,923
Malarial fevers	115,415	1,333	274,053	2,603
Eruptive fevers**	44,438	2,274	38,888	2,050
Dysentery/diarrhea	226,825	3,354	482,764	6,040
Pulmonary diseases	42,204	7,972	19,567	4,607
Rheumatism	29,334	0	88,475	122

*From the beginning of the war to December 31, 1862.
** Eruptive fevers included measles, smallpox, scarlet fever, and erysipelas.

Source: Modified from Medical and Surgical History of the Civil War, *vol. 5, Joseph E. Barnes, ed., surgeon general, U.S. Army.*

Since the number of soldiers in the Union and Confederate armies differed, the number of soldiers wounded and killed or who died from disease as a percentage of the total fighting force will give a more meaningful picture. Thus, annual rates for the number of cases and deaths were from two to three times higher for the Confederate troops than for the Federal forces, except for rheumatism. During the same time period these diseases struck the Union forces fighting in Missouri at annual rates adjusted for strength similar to those for other Federal troops; 25,045 cases of malarial fever with 122 deaths, 25,006 cases of diarrhea or dysentery with 166 deaths, 13,682 cases of pulmonary diseases with 368 deaths and 5,809 cases of eruptive fevers with 162 deaths. Statistics for Confederate soldiers in Missouri are incomplete, but, judging from Union data, very likely annual rates adjusted for strength would be comparable to the entire Confederate forces.

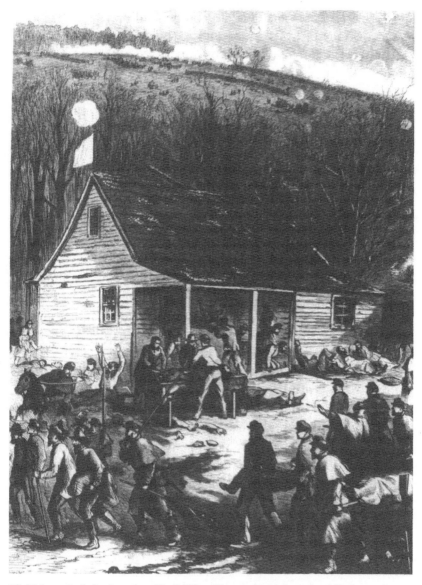

Field hospital during the Civil War. Since physicians had little understanding of sepsis in wounds, having the hospital outside was fortunate. (State Historical Society of Missouri, Columbia)

After careful analysis, the surgeon general and consulting surgeons concluded that inferior equipment as well as a severe shortage of food and clothing resulted in more disease and deaths among Confederate troops than Union forces.

These statistics identify the diseases of consequence at that time, and the comparative mortality rates show the more serious ones, due mainly to the lack of drugs to prevent or treat them. Soldiers and doctors who survived the war learned a valuable lesson about the effects of overcrowding, deficient diet, and poor sanitation. After the war, medical scholars and practicing physicians used the knowledge gained to bring about changes in many medical practices, which improved health care for civilians and for soldiers in later wars. The lessons learned by the military can best be measured by contrasting hospital admission rates in 1861–1862 (Civil War) with those in 1917–1918 (World War I). Admissions for fevers and specific diseases of the intestine (including dysentery and diarrhea) in the Civil War were 29 times higher and the death rate was 258 times higher than during World War I. Since new drugs were not yet available in 1917, sanitation and diet, reinforced by an understanding of the role of microorganisms, accounted for improved conditions.

Soldiers in the Civil War feared disease more than battle; disease caused five times more deaths than did wounds. The impact of disease and the high risk of death from wounds can be seen from a comparison with more recent conflicts in table 2. The information is significant for understanding the suffering of Missourians during the Civil War.

Postwar Missouri was soon attacked by an old enemy. In 1866, another cholera epidemic struck St. Louis. Then the disease appeared in Kansas City. In *One Hundred Years of Medicine and Surgery in Missouri,* Max Goldstein points out that the leaders in Kansas City benefited from the experience gained in the 1849 epidemic in St. Louis. Upon hearing that a man with cholera had gotten off a boat from St. Louis, Kansas City officials ordered a quarantine. Businesses were closed, and citizens had to remain off the streets. Not reassured by this swift action, most inhabitants fled. No more than 400 remained in the city; of those, more than 200 died. Only

Table 2.   *Death from Diseases versus from Wounds* *

Conflict	Disease	Wound
Mexican	102.0	12.9
Civil	62.0	13.3
WWI	25.6	6.1
WWII	16.5	8.1
Korean	0.6	4.5
Vietnam	0.5	2.5

* Numbers are per 100,000 soldiers.

Source: Modified from Civil War Medicine, *Stewart Brooks.*

one doctor stayed to treat the patients, Dr. I. W. Ridge, and he eventually came down with cholera. He sent his hired man to seek the services of a physician in Kansas. Shortly, Dr. Robert Johnson appeared and stayed with Dr. Ridge for two days and two nights. He told his colleague: "Maybe the medicine will take hold on you. If it does, you'll live. But if it doesn't, you will die."

Dr. Ridge survived to practice in Kansas City for twelve more years. Dr. Johnson returned to his practice in Kansas and was elected the first governor of Kansas.

5

Buying a Medical License

Education in Missouri led most advances during the second half of the nineteenth century. The legislature chartered Christian College in Columbia in January 1851. Christian College of Canton, later Culver-Stockton, was incorporated in 1853, and Westminster College, in Fulton, received a charter the same year. Eliot Seminary, founded in 1851, received its charter in February 1853. The founders renamed it Washington Institute in 1854 and Washington University in 1856. Stephens College, incorporated as Columbia Female Baptist College, opened in 1857.

With the help of the federal Morrill Act of 1862, establishing land-grant colleges, and the leadership of Gov. Joseph W. McClurg, the state made substantial progress in providing public higher education after the Civil War. Realizing the need for education for blacks after the war, the men of the Sixty-second and Sixty-fifth Colored Infantries founded Lincoln Institute in Jefferson City in 1866.

The Morrill Act enabled the University of Missouri to establish a College of Agriculture in Columbia and the School of Mines and Metallurgy in Rolla, the area of the state where settlers had originally been drawn by rich mineral deposits. The School of Mines opened in 1870, becoming one of the first technological institutions in the nation and the first west of the Mississippi. The same year Governor McClurg approved an act providing for a "normal school system" in Missouri. The Central State Teachers College opened in Warrensburg in 1871, and the Southwest State Teachers College at Cape Girardeau in 1873. In 1887 college classes began at Lincoln Institute, and in 1890, under the terms of the second Morrill Act, Lincoln became a land-grant college.

For a frontier state with a small population this interest in education was remarkable. An increase in schools granting degrees in medicine soon followed the progress in general education. From 1841 to 1870, forty-four medical schools had been established in Missouri (compared with forty-five in New York and forty-four in Illinois). Many existed but a short time, and by 1876, there were sixty-two regular medical schools plus eleven homeopathic and four eclectic schools in the entire United States. Allopathic doctors practiced much as doctors today do, treating diseases by giving medicines that counteracted the disease. Physicians trained in homeopathy, a system founded by German physician Dr. Samuel Hahneman, used small amounts of drugs that caused signs and symptoms similar to the disease being treated. Eclectic practitioners gave a single specific medicine for a group of symptoms without rendering a diagnosis. For example, they treated menstrual cramps by a tincture of cactus, ground cactus soaked in alcohol and filtered. Osteopathy advanced the concept that structural derangement, especially in the spine, was an important underlying cause of disease and manipulation the best treatment.

During the early years of medical schools, some students received degrees after one or two years of medical training. Others got degrees by training with a doctor in practice without benefit of formal education. For all, there were no standard premedical education requirements. Thus formally educated physicians and those trained by working physicians made up the majority. But some "doctors" simply bought their medical degrees. Little wonder the patient had a difficult time distinguishing the bona fide physician from the quack. In addition, honest differences in philosophies of medical treatment existed. Given the ignorance of the cause of diseases at the time, this is understandable.

In 1855 the board of St. Louis Medical College voted to sever relations with St. Louis University. Although the public assumed the rift was caused by a difference in beliefs between Protestant board members and the Catholic university, the real issue was the simmering conflict between science and religion. The legislature granted St. Louis Medical School an independent charter.

The University of Missouri board of curators discontinued the

Missouri Medical School in St. Louis in 1872 and approved a medical school in Columbia. It opened in 1873 as a two-year school and had fifteen students at a time when the university had 401 undergraduates. In 1891 the medical school expanded to three years of instruction and in 1899 to four.

Both the Kansas Medical College and the College of Physicians and Surgeons opened in Kansas City in 1869. By 1880 the two had joined to establish Kansas City Medical College. The Kansas City University medical department was started at Twelfth and McGee Streets in 1881 and subsequently moved to Tenth and Campbell. Women's Medical College in Kansas City opened in 1895 for the purpose of training more female physicians and remained in existence for eighteen years.

In 1874, Dr. Andrew Still, after years of study into the cause of disease and its cure, abandoned the use of drugs in his practice and became an osteopath. Dr. Still, the son of a preacher, was born in Jonesboro, Virginia, in 1828. As an adult, he moved with his family to Kansas, where he practiced medicine and developed the concept of nerve compression as the cause of disease and advocated treatment by manipulation, theories physicians of traditional medicine disputed. He settled in Macon County, Missouri, to practice osteopathic medicine, and in 1884 the state granted a charter for the American School of Osteopathy.

There was a serious need for better medical care in the state. In April 1883 legislators passed the Medical Practice Act. It required "physicians" who did not hold medical diplomas or certificates from recognized medical schools to sit for an examination administered by the newly established state board of health. Furthermore, to be a recognized school of medicine, a school had to have a regular charter with minimum requirements for curriculum and qualifications for instructors. Surprisingly, it was not until 1894 that the state imposed a medical school entrance requirement: a high school diploma.

The first school of nursing was opened in Boston in 1872 by several women physicians. America's first trained nurse, Linda Richards, graduated October 1, 1873, from North East Hospital for Women and Children in Boston. Schools opened in New York

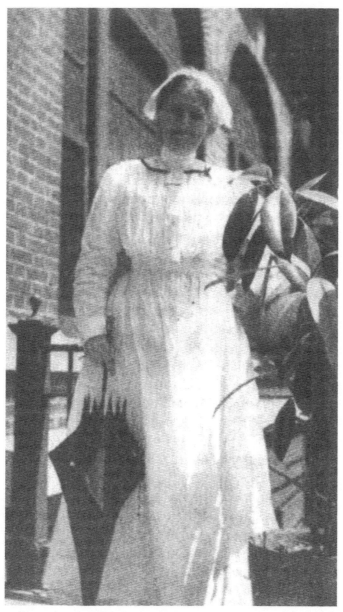

Emma Warr, a native of New York City and a graduate of the New York Hospital Training School for Nurses, became known as Missouri's own "Florence Nightingale." (Missouri Nurses Association, Jefferson City, courtesy State Historical Society of Missouri, Columbia)

and New Haven as well. Emma Warr was the first superintendent of the St. Louis Training School for Nurses, which graduated its first four nurses on April 26, 1886. The improving status of women in society greatly affected the stature gained by nursing in the health-care field.

In the September 22, 1883, *Journal of the American Medical Association,* Dr. E. W. Shauffler of Kansas City reported on the progress of medical and sanitary legislation in Missouri: The law passed at the March 29, 1883, legislative session provided for a board of health to consist of seven members, five to be physicians. The board would have general supervision over "health and sanitary interests of citizens of the state." The board would recommend laws to the general assembly; establish quarantines; give public notice of diseases being epidemic; supervise registration of births, deaths, and vital and mortuary statistics, and require physicians to register names with the county clerk and report all births and deaths within thirty days. The legislature appropriated six thousand dollars to support the act.

In 1884 Dr. E. H. Gregory served as president of the Missouri State Medical Association. He became president of the American Medical Association in 1886. Born in Hopkinsville, Kentucky, in 1824, Gregory studied medicine under Dr. F. W. C. Thomas of Boonville, practiced in Morgan County briefly, and then received a medical degree from St. Louis University Medical Department in 1849. He was professor of surgery in the medical department of Washington University for fifty years and became active in the American Surgical Association, the academic surgeons' society. Minutes of that group's meetings reveal the reluctance with which some physicians accepted medical advances. By this time, the surgeons of the United States were well aware of Joseph Lister's convincing work on use of antisepsis during operations to prevent infections. At the 1884 meeting, held in the Hall of the National Museum Building in Washington, D.C., Gregory commented on a research paper given by Dr. Nicolas Sims, which concluded that practicing aseptic technique to keep away disease-producing microorganisms and using catgut sutures during surgery were safest and most reliable:

I am perhaps an old foggy, for I am not prepared to abandon silk sutures . . . perhaps I was too old when Listerianism came into existence; certainly I have not become enthusiastic on the subject, and I do not know why I have not taken the contagion, because it has prevailed generally. . . . But I cannot attach the same importance to it that some men seem to attach to it.

In 1885 the board of health issued a recommendation that, due to the menace of cholera, county and town boards of health be organized for the safety and protection of their communities. By the end of the nineteenth century the legislature, through the board of health, had become very active, attempting to assure the health of the state's citizens. A handful of physicians worked to improve the ethics and quality of physicians through improved medical education. Unregulated issuance of medical degrees through the many schools in the state continued, and care by physicians, in the absence of scientific explanations of diseases, offered comfort and some relief from pain but few cures.

6

Medical Lessons from War

John C. Gunn in *Gunn's New Domestic Physician or Home Book of Health,* published in 1858, offered the Missouri citizen and soldier then-current medical understanding of diseases. He wrote that fever is "the most common complaint to which the human body is subject" and divided fevers into six groups: (1) inflammatory, (2) intermittent or ague, (3) yellow, (4) remittent, (5) bilious, and (6) nervous or typhus. Apparently, many medical writers described so many types because doctors could not diagnose the cause of most symptoms or diseases. Physicians gave Sappington's "anti-fever" medicine without knowing the cause of the fever. And most physicians still used calomel to purge the "bad humors" from the system.

Common bacteria led to the high mortality in the Civil War: 12.9 per 100,000 wounded, compared with 2.5 deaths per 100,000 wounded in the Korean War. Physicians did not clean amputation saws of blood and tissue from one case to the next; at best they sloshed them in a tub of water teeming with bacteria from previous infected cases. Fortunately, tetanus was a rare complication of wounds, with only 505 cases reported for the entire Union army, because the mortality for tetanus was 89.3 percent. Data is not available for Confederate troops.

Stewart Brooks summarized the status of medicine in *Civil War Medicine:* "For all intended purposes, the doctors and apothecaries of the 1860s knew scarcely more about drugs than did the physician and priests of ancient times."

The minié ball accounted for 94 percent of the wounds and the shell, or canister, for 6 percent. Less then 1,000 soldiers died of saber or bayonet wounds. Over the four years of the war, 44,239 Union soldiers died in battle, and 49,205 more later died of their wounds. Wounds that penetrated the abdomen or the head killed 90 percent of victims, and wounds to the chest, 60 percent.

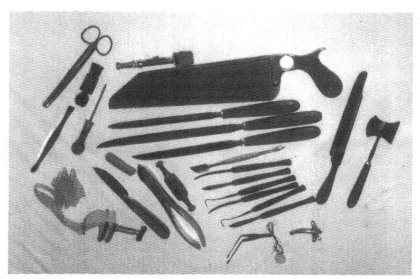

Amputation kit used in the Civil War. The amputation saw was used most frequently (about 29,000 times). Two kits were given to "Doc" Imes by Dr. Lane Brewer when he joined her in Ridgeway for medical practice. The kits were found in a well near Ashland, Kentucky, where they had been hidden when Confederate soldiers overran the farm. (courtesy Mrs. Elvin C. Imes)

As mentioned earlier in the book, amputations were required for the most serious wounds to extremities, or arms and legs. During the war, there were the 174,200 wounds of the extremities. Records show that 7,096 soldiers died from the 29,980 amputations. The higher up the leg the surgeon had to amputate, the more likely the patient was to die: 6 percent of soldiers who had a foot removed died. For those whose amputation was at the ankle, 25 percent died; and at mid-thigh, 58 percent. Amputation of the hip resulted in an 83 percent mortality. In comparing deaths in the Confederate army with those of the Federal troops for the four years, strength of forces is important; the Union forces totaled slightly more than four million, while the Confederate numbered approximately 1.2 million. Further, military experts point out many discrepancies in Confederate reports. Nevertheless, the records show that 52,954

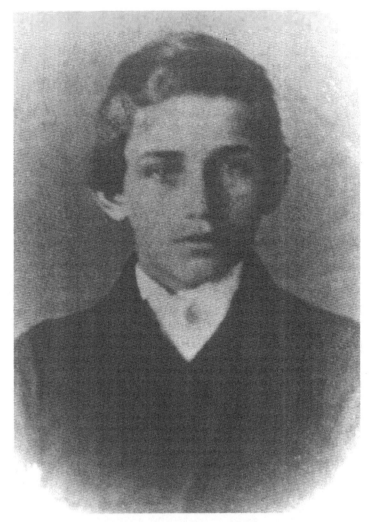

Caspar Geisberg of Jefferson City went to St. Louis in May 1861 and enlisted in the Eighth Illinois Regiment. At the Battle of Fort Donelson in February 1862, a shell smashed his left arm, and he got a deep wound in his leg. Friends dragged him to a log cabin, where he lost consciousness and his feet and right hand were affected by the frost. On the third day, doctors in Dover amputated his arm, and he was hospitalized in Mound City. His uncle, Dr. Bernard Bruns, mayor of Jefferson City, saw his name on the list of wounded and went to get him. They traveled by steamer from Cairo, rested in St. Louis, and finally reached Jefferson City. On March 18, four days after returning home, he died. (A. E. Schroeder collection)

Confederates were killed in battle, and an additional 32,570 died later from their wounds. The second number is probably too low. During the same time, Union forces suffered 186,216 deaths from disease and Confederate troops had 59,277 deaths from disease.

Whether by luck or miracle, some soldiers survived. The story told to Ray Dankenbring, an author living in St. Louis, reveals perhaps the true picture of the role of army surgeons in treating abdominal wounds: "My great grandmother found her son floating in a stream. His belly had been slashed and some guts were hanging out. She treated him and he survived." Without major bleeding or holes in the intestine, he had a better chance of escaping fatal peritonitis, an infection in the abdomen, by receiving treatment out of the hospital setting away from the grossly contaminated instruments used by surgeons.

The medical profession itself suffered some losses during the Civil War, though not many from wounds inflicted by the enemy during battle. In one recorded case, the Confederates at Pilot Knob wounded a Dr. Pollack and took him prisoner. Federal forces arrested Dr. Sidney Robinson in Versailles, where he had gone to attend a sick grandchild, and hanged him as a Southern sympathizer. Union troops sentenced and shot Dr. Thomas S. Foster when he was caught after burning a bridge over the Salt River. A doctor referred to only by his last name, Murphy, who had amputated the arm of a Mr. Taylor, was arrested at Ewing's farm, but finally released. Perhaps the successful amputation saved both the patient and the doctor.

The reports of the physicians examining recruits for the army contain interesting information about the general health of Missourians at the time of the Civil War. Included in the *U.S. Provost-Marshall General's Bureau Report* is an extract of notes made by Dr. James R. McCormick from the third district in southeast Missouri.

On May 30, 1865, in Ironton, McCormick wrote:

> Inflammatory fevers are more active, and in this the treatment of blood-letting is more frequently demanded, in the mountaineer country than in the swamp districts. . . . Typhoid fever made its appearance in southeast Missouri about ten years ago. . . . During the last four years it has increased in frequency and intensity.

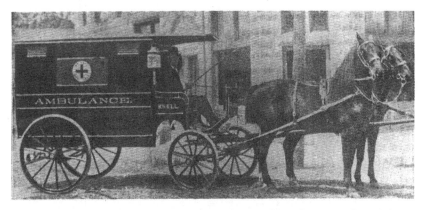

Horse drawn ambulance. Covered wagons and carriages replaced the flatbed wagons used as ambulances early in the war. (State Historical Society of Missouri, Columbia)

In performing 732 physical examinations, McCormick had found tuberculosis, the most common cause of exemption, in 52 men. Hernias were present in 33. The condition was present in one out of ten men over the age of 21, and a marked increase of hernia occurred in men over age 45. This suggests that the majority of troops were 21 years of age or younger. The poor health of the general citizenry explains, in part, why so many died of disease during the war. This picture helps us understand why the average life expectancy in the 1800s was 45 years.

Slowly, throughout the nineteenth century, the medical profession gained a scientific understanding of human physiology and pathology so that physicians had a more sophisticated basis for diagnosing diseases. But the drugs and procedures to treat diseases lagged behind these advances.

Home remedies were still being listed by the *Jefferson City Tribune,* on May 17, 1871: "For sore throat beat white of two eggs with two teaspoons of white sugar and add a pint of lukewarm water; grate a little nutmeg into a mixture, stir, and drink frequently."

Researchers have found evidence of cancer in an Egyptian mummy. Given the inability of physicians to cure many simpler diseases even thousands of years later, one would expect a suggested home remedy for cancer. In the April 12, 1871, issue of the *Tribune* just such a concoction is described: "Break an egg, retaining the yolk. Add salt and stir until a salve is formed. Place a portion on a piece of sticking plaster and apply two times a day."

For treating sunstroke, one dissolved salt in tepid water and poured it into the patient's ears. The treatment of corns required the person to use one teaspoon of tar, one teaspoon of coarse brown sugar, and one of saltpeter, warm them together and then after spreading the concoction on kid leather, place it on the spot. In two days this was supposed to draw out the corns.

On July 11, 1878, a traveler from New Orleans, William P. O'Bannon, was diagnosed with the first confirmed case of yellow fever in St. Louis. C. W. Francis, the health commissioner of St. Louis, promptly opened a quarantine hospital with Dr. Harvey C. Davis as superintendent. O'Bannon died on July 19. In 1878, thirty-three out of seventy-one patients with yellow fever died, and in 1879 four out of thirty-five.

Although cholera had disappeared, and a vaccine had become available for smallpox, other diseases struck the state. The common viral and bacterial diseases—diphtheria, scarlet fever (streptococcus), and tuberculosis—went unchecked. "Croup" could have been from a virus or whooping cough. Today there are antibiotics to fight these diseases, but physicians then had none. Table 3, compiled by Dr. Walter B. Dorsett, clearly shows the status of contagious diseases in the late 1800s.

This table suggests that the efforts to improve the water and sewer systems produced results. Population figures help put these numbers in perspective; St. Louis had 70,860 inhabitants in 1850 and 568,000 in 1896.

The nineteenth century ended with increased recognition of the environmental factors that impose a risk to health. Regulations relating to community health and collecting vital statistics proved a sound foundation for improvement. Although standards of physician education and practice were inadequate, attempts to set new standards indicated the state's leaders recognized the need for improvement.

As the century ended, the medical profession still had few cures

Table 3. *Cases of Contagious Diseases in St. Louis*
1850-1896

Year	Small-pox	Diph-theria	Typhoid fever	Scarlet fever	*Croup/ Consump.	Cholera
1850	7	0	125	0	865	4,210
1867	18	48	194	27	522	3,002
1872	1591	76	176	47	665	1
1886	1	889	124	149	1,075	131
1888-1889	4	149	99	25	1,130	0
1893-1894	1	198	171	55	1,117	0
1895-1896	24	526	100	18	1,163	0

* "Croup" and "Consumptive cough" have been combined.

Source: One Hundred Years of Medicine and Surgery in Missouri, *Max A. Goldstein.*

to offer, save for quinine and smallpox vaccine. Indeed, they had virtually no aids or ability to render specific diagnoses. Understanding the role bacteria played in disease plus the discovery of anesthesia and antisepsis was to catapult medicine into the twentieth century.

Part III

Standards for Medicine 1899–1948

Medical Education in Missouri is at a low ebb . . . six medical schools are utterly wretched . . .
—*Abraham Flexner,* Medical Education in the United States and Canada, *1912*

Introduction

The Missouri and Mississippi Rivers were still important alternatives for the transportation of goods, especially grain and minerals, in the 1900s. Construction of levees and dams enhanced safety for barges and controlled flooding to some degree. But as towns sprang up away from river access, a network of railroads developed, and with the increasing use of automobiles and trucks, roads became important. The telephone came to the rural Ozarks about 1910, providing better communication. Congress created the Rural Electrification Administration in 1935, but by 1940 fewer than one in five farms in Missouri had electricity.

Throughout the United States, medicine benefited from the increased availability of information about the different state regulations for health officials and professional practice as well as the educational and ethical requirements for hospitals and physicians. And still the existence of large numbers of physicians who lacked solid credentials prompted Henry S. Pritchett, president of the Carnegie Foundation for the Advancement of Teaching, to ask Abraham Flexner to conduct a national survey of medical schools. From 1908 to 1910, Flexner visited the nation's medical schools. The report of his findings radically changed medical education and the relationship of education to the practice of medicine. But while science helped doctors to understand and diagnose disease, it offered meager aid for treating ailments.

Two world wars and an economic depression absorbed the U.S. for almost fifty years. From 1899 to 1948, industrial advances quickly changed the nation and Missouri from a mostly agricultural society to an industrial and urban society, bringing new health risks. Local and state governments struggled with the problems created by expansion of cities that outstripped community planning.

Easier travel for citizens meant more rapid spread of viral diseases, as demonstrated by the flu epidemic of World War I. Unlike the diseases of the Civil War, the flu that hit the army, causing a huge number of hospital admissions, spread rapidly to the civilian population in the United States. There was a deadly viral epidemic, and the young and infirm who caught the flu frequently died from a secondary infection, pneumonia. Cary Haynes of Kansas City was born and raised on a farm near Richmond, Missouri, during World War I. Her father contracted the flu and barely survived. She recalled, "Others weren't so lucky. A lot of people died at that time."

During this period there was a significant development in education. Many medical schools closed due to new strict requirements on faculty and curriculum. Scientific advances led to better understanding of the basis of most diseases, which allowed communities to enact important health laws and improved the diagnostic ability of physicians. Specialization of medical practice began, but because there were still few cures, most Missourians grew up without ever seeing a physician.

For many, visits to the doctor occurred only when injuries had to be treated. Tom Arnold, a retired attorney from Benton, saw a doctor once while growing up. "I cut my finger on a knife, a Christmas present, and Doctor Wade sewed the laceration together." Cary Haynes said the only time she saw a doctor was as a four-year-old child. The doctor stitched a gash on her forehead.

Tom Arnold's grandfather, Marshall, was an attorney in Iron County during the late 1800s. "He died in 1913 of tuberculosis. The only treatment he received was a brew of hickory-tobacco

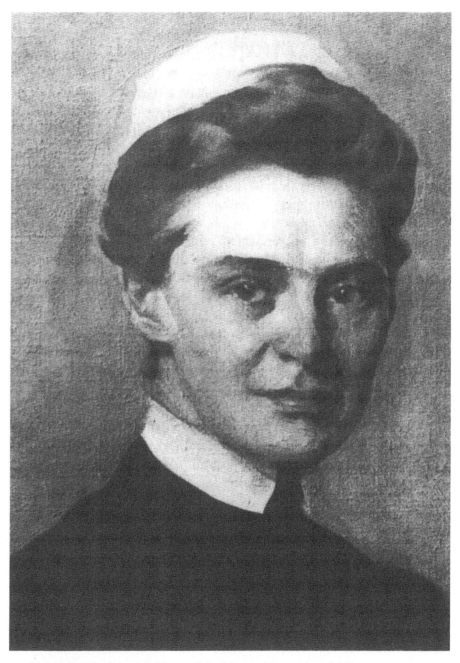

Isabel Robb, first president of the Nurses' Associated Alumnae.
(Lowell Press, Kansas City)

leaves. No medicines existed at that time for tuberculosis," Arnold explained.

Ray Dankenbring was raised near Sweet Springs. In the late 1930s, his brother developed diphtheria. When his throat closed and he was dying, the family doctor made a slash with a penknife and put a straw through the hole. The young boy breathed through the straw and is still alive; he's now eighty years old. However, when his father contracted tuberculosis, like Marshall Arnold, he received no medicine. Ray recalled those days. "He slept in a tent in the back yard for six months. Pretty crude isolation," he said. In the absence of antibiotics quarantine was a routine procedure in the early nineteenth century.

Bob Blaine, who also grew up on a farm near Richmond during this era, recalled that he and his sister got all the childhood diseases and never saw a physician. Coal oil was the family panacea for almost any ailment. When his father got diphtheria, the county health officer put a pink sign, a quarantine sign, on their house. Elaine Simerly also remembers the pink sign that appeared on the house when diphtheria struck her family. Fumigation of the house soon followed, forcing the family to sleep in the haymow. Frequently, at the end of the quarantine period, county health officials fumigated the house by burning a sulfur candle.

Health agencies were diligent in using quarantine to control contagious diseases for which no effective treatments were available, especially those that carried a significant risk of death: erysipelas, diphtheria, and measles had a death rate of 5 to 10 percent, with the very young being most likely to die. Smallpox and tuberculosis had death rates from 20 to 40 percent, with the young, the old, and those in poor health having the higher death rates. The same groups were also more likely to die of pneumonia, which killed about 25 percent of victims. Yet families rarely called physicians except for injuries or in desperation, as with Dankenbring's brother; without effective drugs, quarantine was the most effective measure.

7

Growth of Travel, Cities, and Medical Schools

The devastating floods of 1843 and 1866, along with yearly problems of varying water levels in the river had led to the construction of dams on the Mississippi River. The Army Corps of Engineers built a dam at Keokuk, Iowa, at the Missouri-Iowa border, between 1910 and 1913. Soon a bridge spanned the river below the dam, replacing one of the busiest ferry crossings, the one at Alexandria. Following the federal government's action in 1917 to assume responsibility for flood control, the corps constructed seven dams and locks, beginning in Keokuk and continuing to just below St. Louis, in an attempt to control flooding. Most were completed by 1939.

While the Mississippi was still used to move goods north and and grain south, by the 1900s railroads had become the popular means of travel. Although roads had replaced the wagon trails of the nineteenth century, using them required a certain degree of daring. For example, after passing through Keokuk, Iowa, the motorist crossed the Des Moines River by driving on planks that straddled the rails of the railroad bridge. Safely on the Missouri side, drivers headed south on Route 61, the old Salt River Road, over a narrow cement highway which had replaced a dirt road that turned to mud in a downpour.

Three miles beyond the railroad bridge sat Alexandria, Missouri. In 1939, I spent the summer, as I had done for years, enjoying the rigors of life on the Jenkins farm, located on Route 61 one mile north of Gregory Road. That year ringworm of the scalp broke out. A thirteen-mile trip in the family auto brought me to a physician's office located in the rear of the only gas station at Alexandria. The gray-haired, bearded physician made the diagnosis, proceeded to

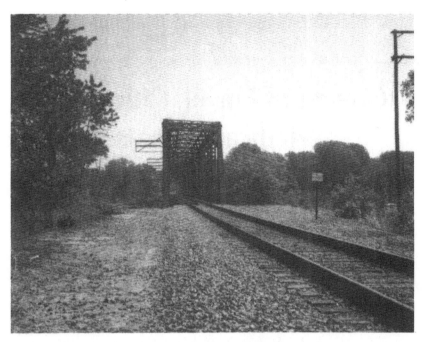

The railroad bridge over the Des Moines River. Travelers ascertained that no trains approached and then cautiously steered the vehicle toward the Missouri side, one observer peering out the left side and another out the right side to help the driver stay on the planks. (photo by the author)

shave my head, and then painted my scalp with gentian violet, a certain cure for the infection at that time. Violet scalps were not the rage in the city so the isolation of the farm was never more welcome.

The wars of the nineteenth and twentieth centuries had distinct differences. The Civil War was fought to some extent in Missouri but largely in the eastern states. Twentieth-century wars were global with no conflict on U.S. soil. During the Civil War, disease killed 62 out of every 1,000 soldiers; in World War I, only 16.5 out of 1,000 died from disease. Twelve out of 1,000 deaths in World War I resulted from pneumonia and flu, a significant problem among civilians as well, as noted above. "If we can eliminate the latter factor [death from flu] in the next war, granting the hypothesis that there is to be a next war, what a good showing we should make." This quote by an editor of the journal *Military Surgeon,* published in 1921, both betrays the suspicion following World War I that another war was inevitable and demonstrates the impact the flu and pneumonia had on troops.

Table 4. *Mortality from Diseases in World War I versus the Civil War*

Disease	WWI–#deaths*	Civil War–# deaths**
Pneumonia	41,747	38,962
Malaria	13	13,951
Diphtheria	100	1,188
Typhoid fever	213	51,133
Scarlet fever	167	1126
Tuberculosis	1,220	9,574
Smallpox	5	9,536
Meningitis	2,137	3,859
Dysentery	42	63,898

* Deaths September 1, 1917 to December 31, 1919.
** Deaths that would have occurred based on death rate of Civil War and same number of soldiers as WWI.

Source: Modified from Military Surgeon, *vol. 48, 1921.*

Further, death from disease in the Civil War was five times more common than from wounds; in comparison an equal rate for diseases and wounds occurred in World War I. In that war 10,385 Missourians were wounded, and 2,562 others died.

Following the formation of the American Nurses Association in 1896, the number of trained nurses had grown rapidly, and more than 24,000, over 25 percent of the graduate nurses in the U.S., served during World War I. Linda Flanagan in *One Strong Voice* defines the status of nursing in 1922 by quoting Clara D. Noyes, president of the American Nurses Association: "The world's war settled, if it needed settling, the question of the position for the nursing profession."

For civilians, the commonest causes of mortality in the United States and their change from 1910 to 1940 is similar to the change in cause of mortality from diseases in the two wars.

Table 5. *Death Rates per 100,000 U.S. Population*

Disease	1915	1920	1930	1940
Pneumonia	130.3	136.8	82.3	54.9
Diarrhea	67.1	53.6	26.0	10.3
Puerperal	14.7	19.0	12.7	7.0
Nephritis	101.5	88.7	91.0	81.5
Motor vehicle accident	5.8	10.3	24.5	26.2

Source: Vital Statistics in the United States 1940-1960: National Center for Health Statistics.

Table 5 reveals changes in health problems for Missouri citizens during this period. Deaths from nephritis dropped somewhat. Before the appearance of penicillin, drugs such as neoprontisil and sulfa were effective for all but the more serious streptococcal infections. The drugs dramatically decreased the death rate from birth infections, diarrhea, and pneumonia. At the same time, deaths from auto accidents increased by five times.

Researchers have compared Missouri's death rate per 100,000 population for all causes with that of the nation. They found that health risks in Missouri were similar to those in the United States in general. The environment was no longer so often the cause of illness, except for auto accidents and rapid spread of viral diseases. Treatments for diseases caused by streptococcus began the era of wonder drugs. Serious infections and infections from bacteria other than streptococcus still posed a high risk to health. Penicillin, the miracle drug, was the first shot in the antibiotic war against bacteria. Dr. Barry Wood Jr. of Barnes Hospital commented on the use of penicillin in the June 27, 1943, issue of the *St. Louis Post-Dispatch,* saying that it was "materially checking

Table 6. *Death Rate per 100,000 Population in 1940*

Cause	Missouri	U.S.
All	1,156.2	1,076.4
Heart, all diseases	296.3	292.6
Cancer	134.1	120.3
Nephritis	112.7	81.5
Influenza	96.6	70.3
CNS/vascular	99.9	90.9
Tuberculosis	46.5	45.9
Acute rheumatic fever	1.0	1.3
Diabetes	25.2	26.2
Motor vehicle accident	22.9	26.2
Syphilis	18.7	14.4

Source: Modified from Vital Statistics in the United States in 1940, Part 2, *U.S. Department of Commerce, Bureau of the Census.*

the growth of staphylococcus bacteria . . . penicillin has been found successful in treating infections caused by pneumococcus and streptococcus bacteria." Staphylococcus, then as now, was everywhere.

Dr. Alexander Fleming of England first noted penicillin, produced by a mold, "penicillium," in 1928. He had grown staphylococcus bacteria on a blood-agar plate to test the effect of chemicals on the bacteria. Several days later, he threw the plates out because a mold was growing amongst the bacteria, contaminating it. Years later, he realized that around the mold the bacteria had been killed. Intensive investigation revealed the mold produced a substance, penicillin, that readily killed streptococcus as well as staphylococcus. Serendipity, the making of a discovery by happenstance, has led to many important innovations. Although Fleming received numerous honors, including the Nobel Prize, for his discovery, he remained a humble, almost shy man. Andre

Maurois in *The Life of Sir Alexander Fleming* tells of Fleming's speech for Harvard's 1945 commencement. Fleming told the audience of his initial observation and the ten-year delay in recognizing its significance. Then several more years passed before physicians had penicillin to prevent thousands of deaths from infections. "There is, then, nothing new in my advice to the young. Work hard, work well, do not clutter up the mind too much with precedents, and be prepared to accept such good fortune as the gods offer."

As Dr. Fleming told the students at Harvard, even after penicillin was discovered, it was not immediately used everywhere. Howard Jenkins was forty-three years old when he got a cut on his great toe during a minor auto accident on the Eads Bridge in 1940. The wound became infected with "staph." He developed blood poisoning and died. Penicillin was not available in Missouri until the mid-forties.

Following the discovery of penicillin, scientists discovered other antibiotics, many active against bacteria not attacked by penicillin. Dr. Hugh E. Stephenson Jr. in *Aesculapius Was a Mizzou Tiger: History of Medicine at Ole Mizzou,* published in 1998, records the great contributions the University of Missouri–Columbia made in the war against bacterial infections. In addition to chemicals, scientists tested a vast number of soil samples. They reasoned that organisms might be found in the wide variety of soils that produced antibiotics effective against bacteria resistant to antibiotics then in use.

Two exciting discoveries came from scientists who had worked in the university's botany department. Dr. Paul R. Brukholder tested soil samples from Venezuela in a laboratory at Yale University. In 1947 he discovered chloramphenicol, a broad-spectrum antibiotic—one that attacks many different species of bacteria—obtained from cultures of *Streptomyces venezuelae.* The drug was called Chloromycetin by the pharmaceutical company and was effective against many bacteria, some viruses, and most rickettsial organisms, bacterialike microorganisms carried by ticks.

Soil samples from Sanborn Field, the experimental field on the University of Missouri–Columbia campus, provided another broad-

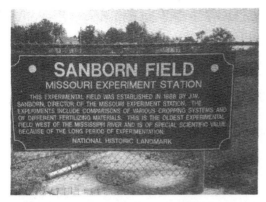 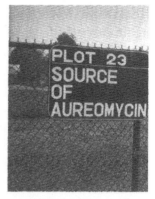

Sanborn Field, located on the University of Missouri–Columbia campus at Rollins Road and College Avenue. Dr. Duggar found aureomycin, the pharmaceutical trademark for chlortetracycline, from a soil sample Dr. Albrecht obtained from the Timothy grass plot. (photo by the author)

spectrum antibiotic. Dr. Wiliam A. Albrecht, chairman of the college's soil department, sent soil samples to his friend Benjamin M. Duggar, who searched for new antibiotics in a lab owned by a drug company—Lederle Laboratories—in Pearl River, New York. Dr. Duggar, who had been head of the university's botany department from 1902 until 1907, isolated aureomycin. Dr. Duggar, then seventy-eight years old, gave the previously unknown species of actinomycetes the name *Streptomyces aureofaciens*. He died six years later from pneumonia, caused by a bacterial strain resistant to aureomycin.

The prevention of contagious diseases had improved dramatically by midcentury, thanks to quarantine and vaccination programs. In 1940, health officials recorded no deaths from cholera. That year, for every 100,000 people in the U.S., typhoid fever caused 1.5 deaths; diphtheria caused 1.1; whooping cough, 2.2; erysipelas (due to streptococcus), 0.3 deaths; and scarlet fever, 0.5 deaths.

Two world wars, the telephone, the radio, and the airplane brought modernization and the beginning of urbanization to

Missouri. In 1940, St. Louis had 816,048 inhabitants and was the eighth-largest city in the United States. The population of Kansas City was 399,178, Joplin, 37,144, St. Joseph, 75,742, and Springfield, the fourth-largest city in Missouri, was 61,238.

Rapid growth created problems for medicine over the next fifty years. Medical care for inner-city and rural Missourians, compared to the rest of the populace, began to deteriorate.

8

Improving Medical Education

General education in Missouri moved ahead as city and county governments established more elementary and high schools throughout the state. In the early 1900s health education was introduced in public schools. Students attending the Gravel Hill School in Clark County, on the corner of Gregory Road and Route 61, before the First World War studied *Introductory Physiology and Hygiene* by H. W. Conn, M.D. The text included twelve "Everyday Health Rules" for a healthy lifestyle:

1. Rise and go to bed early.
2. Eat good nourishing food.
3. Drink plenty of fresh, clean water.
4. Let tobacco and alcohol alone.
5. Work while you work and cheerfully.
6. Play when you play and heartily.
7. Get plenty of exercise, stay out of doors, especially in winter.
8. Keep lungs active with long breaths.
9. Exercise skin with cold baths and rubbing.
10. Do not wear tight clothing of any kind.
11. Be sure the rooms you live and sleep in are well ventilated.
12. Train yourself to be the skillful engineer of your body's engine. Be ambitious to possess a strong, healthy and graceful body.

The legislature authorized more teachers colleges, located strategically throughout the state. This progress in general education produced better applicants for medical schools that groaned under pressure to improve. St. Louis University purchased the Marion Sims–Beaumont Medical College in 1903 for its school of medicine.

In 1906 the directors of Washington University renamed their

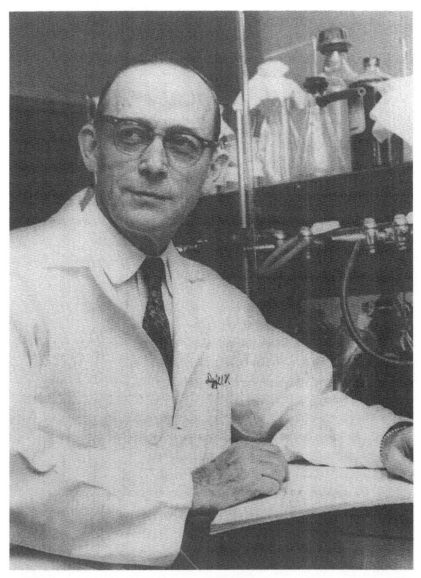

Dr. Warren H. Cole, codiscoverer of the first test to diagnose diseased gallbladders using x-rays. In 1936 he left St. Louis to take the chair of surgery at the University of Illinois School of Medicine in Chicago, where he developed an outstanding surgery training program and continued his research interest, switching to cancer research in the 1940s. (photo by the author)

medical school "the Medical Department of Washington University" and incorporated it into the university. A trust established in 1892 by Robert Barnes, a St. Louis wholesale grocer and banker, had left a large sum for a hospital. In 1915 the board of directors determined that the medical department should become a private academic institution. That year, Barnes Hospital, which was to be Washington University's primary teaching hospital, finally opened after repeated delays. Soon, important discoveries by faculty researchers rewarded the university. Two Washington University physicians, Dr. Warren Cole and Dr. Evarts Graham discovered the test to diagnose gallbladder disease in a Barnes Hospital research laboratory. In 1933 Dr. Graham, the chairman of surgery at Washington University, was the first physician in the U.S. to successfully remove a patient's lung.

Following the establishment of the American School of Osteopathy in Kirksville in 1892, the discipline expanded steadily, and by 1937 there were osteopathic schools in Kansas City, Des Moines, Los Angeles, Chicago, and Philadelphia. Osteopathic graduates began to receive specialty training in pediatrics, obstetrics and gynecology, internal medicine, and surgery. The emphasis on manipulation as the primary form of treatment diminished, allowing osteopathic physicians to sit for the same state licensing exam as those taken by medical school graduates.

In 1909 the University of Missouri School of Medicine at Columbia reverted to a two-year school since faculty did not have enough patients to train medical students in their two clinical years. The university began to award bachelor's degrees in medicine to their students, who then transferred to other schools for two years of clinical instruction.

By 1908 the United States had 148 medical schools with 22,148 enrollees and an income from fees of $2,729,251. Medical training was still by preceptor, a physician who trained students by taking them into his practice, or often by quacks who passed on superstitions. Kansas City's schools were diploma mills, giving degrees to anyone, until 1923. That year a reporter from the *Kansas City Journal Post* walked into the Kansas City College of Medicine and Surgery at 2225 Holmes Street, paid money, and, without attending a class or receiving any form of training, got a medical certificate. When he revealed how easy it had been, the revelation forced change.

Like other states, Missouri needed standards of medical education. In 1894 the Missouri legislature had passed a bill requiring at least a high school education for admission to medical school. In 1920 the legislators increased the requirements to become a doctor: a college degree for admission plus a four-year medical curriculum and a year's internship were necessary to be licensed in the state. Students also had to pass a written and clinical examination.

The survey of medical schools by Abraham Flexner changed the face of medicine drastically. In 1912 he had reported his findings in *Medical Education in the United States and Canada.* He found 1,780 students enrolled in 13 schools in Missouri. The American School of Osteopathy in Kirksville (560), the St. Louis School of Medicine (243), the St. Louis College of Physicians and Surgeons (244), and the University Medical College in Kansas City, which was not associated with the University of Missouri (174), had the largest enrollments. In his report, Flexner concluded, "medical education in Missouri is at a low ebb. . . . six schools are utterly wretched and four without promise. . . . the State Board of Healing Arts lacks authority to enforce requirements."

Some of Flexner's solutions solved the problem of too many medical schools and, more important, they forced standards of medical education to greatly improve. Missouri heeded the message. By 1938, the number of medical schools had dropped to three.

Missouri was the first state west of the Mississippi River to establish a state cancer hospital. Health officials and physicians sensed a mounting problem from the increasing death rate from cancer. In 1920, the death rate from all cancers was 74.5 per 100,000 people. By 1930, the rate had risen to 108 per 100,000. In that time, the population had increased by 6.6 percent, but the number of people dying from cancer had increased by 54.3 percent.

Dr. Ellis Fischel of St. Louis initially did not want Missouri to

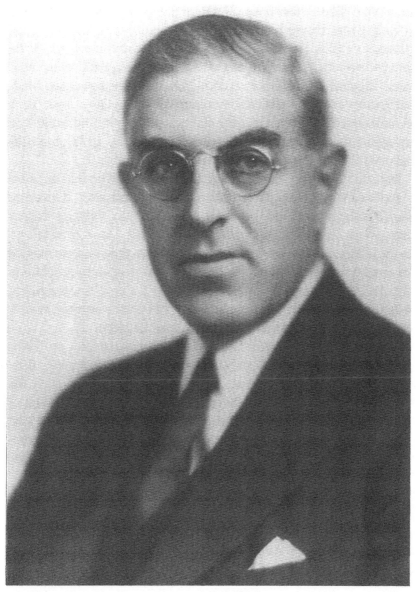

Dr. Ellis Fischel served on the cancer commission. Perhaps his strong belief that a statewide cancer program should be established changed his opinion about a state cancer hospital. Some thought it due to the persuasion of Gov. Lloyd Stark and the opportunity for Fischel to pull together his experience as a surgeon, his dedicated service to suffering humanity, and his talent as an organizer. (Ellis Fischel Hospital)

establish a state cancer hospital. Other physicians had reservations as well. Craig Doyle reported in his thesis for a master's degree, "History of Ellis Fischel," the feelings of several members of the medical society: "The hospital will be the wedge for state medicine." Regardless of these reservations, the Missouri State Medical Society established a cancer commission, and Gov. Lloyd Stark recommended to the legislature that a state hospital be built. The groundbreaking ceremony took place August 29, 1938, and officials laid the cornerstone in Columbia on December 9.

Ironically, the governor appointed Dr. Fischel, who had opposed a state cancer hospital, to the cancer commission. Governor Stark's enthusiasm and his own dedication to fighting cancer changed Dr. Fischel's feelings about the project. He worked relentlessly as the commission's chairman and more than anyone pushed the project forward. Tragically, he was killed in an auto accident in May 1938 on Route 63 while on his way to a commission meeting in Jefferson City. Dr. Fischel never saw his dream become reality. Dedication of the hospital took place April 26, 1940.

But long before a cancer hospital could open, several problems had to be solved: location, private versus state run, private or indigent patients, and the system for controlling the hospital were the major issues. In the end, the hospital was located in the middle of the state and was used for indigent cancer patients, those who could not pay for their care. Control was to rest with the governor through the Missouri Cancer Commission, and he would select the four members of the commission.

Dr. Lauren Ackerman, a graduate of the University of Rochester Medical School in New York, served as the first hospital medical director and pathologist. His view that "Departments must have equal strength" was a visionary one and resulted in the first multidisciplinary management of cancer in the United States.

The first surgeon in chief, Dr. Eugene Bricker, stayed only six months. After he left to join the army, Dr. Everett D. Sugarbaker replaced him. A graduate of Cornell Medical School in New York, Dr. Sugarbaker had extensive surgical training, two years of internship, one year of training for bowel surgery, and then six months at the tumor clinic of the National Cancer Institute. He

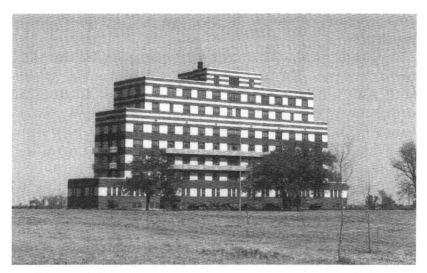

Ellis Fischel Hospital soon after its completion. (State Historical
Society of Missouri, Columbia)

was the first surgeon west of the Mississippi River to have special
training in cancer surgery. To counter the undercurrent of anxiety
about Ellis Fischel being the wedge for state medicine, he method-
ically went about the state talking to medical groups, reassuring
physicians that the hospital existed to help them manage their indigent cancer patients. Still, Dr. Sugarbaker recalled, at a dinner
preceding one of his talks, a physician asked, "Are you a commu-
nist, Dr. Sugarbaker?"

Dr. Theodore P. Eberhard led the third department, radiation
therapy. Like Bricker, he left after six months for the army. Dr.
Juan A. del Regato replaced him. Dr. del Regato had gone to medical school in Paris and was recognized as one of the leading radiation therapists in the United States. He stayed at Ellis Fischel.

In 1944, 1,171 new patients visited the hospital for outpatient
care. Total visits to the clinic were 5,576. New in-patient admissions to the hospital that year were 1,013, plus the readmission of
605 established patients. While the hospital was never as successful as other famous cancer hospitals in the U.S., like Memorial
Hospital in New York City or M. D. Anderson in Houston, it did

serve the cancer patients of the state who could not afford private treatment.

Many other improvements took place during the first half of the twentieth century. The state board of health set hospital requirements, and the board of healing arts instituted medical school and physician standards. Backed by an enlightened legislature, the environment for a healthier citizenry steadily improved; vital statistics showed the death rate for those under 45 years of age as well as those over 65 decreased between 1920 and 1940. In 1939–1941, the average life expectancy was 62.8 for males and 67.3 for females.

After World War I nurses grew in both visibility and in the scope of care they rendered. They were the hands-on caregivers, and soon replaced the next-door neighbor in giving care at the scene of injuries and delivery of babies. Shortly after Mary Faurot was born in Hannibal, where her grandfather was a successful physician, her parents moved to North Dakota. Since they lived on a ranch several miles from Bismarck and the nearest doctor, her mother moved into town when she was almost ready to deliver Mary's sister Rose. Unfortunately, when her labor began they found that the doctor had gone by train to a nearby town to see a sick patient. Since the next train wasn't due until the following day, he started for Bismarck on a handcar, an unusual form of travel for the country doctor of the early 1900s. He arrived too late. A nurse delivered Rose, an example of the coming role of nursing as well as an indication of the obstacles faced by patients and physicians who lived "in the country."

9

Scientific Diagnosis

The discovery of the x-ray in 1895 had revolutionized diagnosis of problems arising in the chest and abdominal cavities and of injuries. Researchers in bacterial science isolated and identified organisms causing infectious diseases so that doctors were able to determine the cause of many of those diseases. Sophisticated advances in physiology led to laboratory tests to determine the function of organs such as the liver, lung, stomach, intestines, heart, and kidney. Surgical procedures used sterile techniques to kill bacteria on anything that might touch the area of the operation.

The discovery of insulin by Frederick Banting and Charles Best in 1936 and penicillin by Sir Alexander Fleming along with the wide use of sulfa drugs by 1940 allowed physicians to move beyond sitting at the bedside of patients all night, able to offer only modest comfort. Cures of diseases, however, except for a few surgical procedures and the ability to save limb and life from trauma, were still rare.

The number of vaccines to prevent disease increased. They began to be used to prevent childhood diseases, and in World War II, every soldier received a tetanus immunization (using tetanus toxoid) to prevent lockjaw. Only six soldiers out of 1,000,000 wounded suffered from lockjaw compared with the World War I rate of 800 per 100,000. And at that, of the fifteen cases of tetanus in WWII, eleven of those developing it had not received tetanus immunization. Field hospitals had better results in World War II than in previous wars. During the war, 83 percent of the wounded who reached the field hospital survived, compared with 22 percent in World War I. Medical personnel sprinkled sulfa in open wounds and aggressively removed dead tissue. The soldiers' immunizations and the use of sterile techniques and antibiotics protected the wounded from infection. After the war, military physicians applied these principles at home to save the lives and limbs of Missourians injured in farm and highway accidents.

The case of the University of Missouri's renowned football coach Don Faurot demonstrates the approach taken to farm or road accidents before the Second World War and the specializations in treatments used afterward. "Coach" was raised on a farm near Mountain Grove, where his father ran a state experimental fruit station. In 1913, at the age of nine, he was with his father, who was spraying trees. The horses pulling the machinery suddenly lurched forward, throwing the young boy into the machinery behind. Luckily, he lost only two fingers at the knuckle. Mary Faurot, his widow, said, "Without those fingers he went on to letter in three sports at the University of Missouri, although he had to get special dispensation to serve in World War Two." She continued, "Today, they would have brought those fingers to the hospital in ice and sewed them back on." Reimplantation of limbs has been successful in a number of cases.

Care of the injured before World War II, whether on the farm, the highways, or the job, was not much different from that given at the time of the Civil War, except for the use of sterile techniques in caring for the wounds.

Francis Haynes was returning from Excelsior Springs one night in 1937. The eighteen-year-old and a high school buddy, who was asleep in the backseat, had been at a party. Francis was driving on a gravel road with his arm out the window when a truck sideswiped their car. He remembers that the impact tore the side of the car apart.

> My dangling arm was bleeding bad. Luckily this happened across the road from a country store. A man at the store who had medical experience in World War I put a tourniquet on the arm and told me to release it every five or ten minutes. Dr. Elmer Gray went in the ambulance on the trip to Kansas City. My friend who was in the back seat had a bad head injury. He died in the ambulance as we went through Excelsior Springs on the way to St. Joe's Hospital, the old one.

In the hospital the night-shift nurse smelled gangrene, and the doctors took Francis to the operating room and amputated his arm.

Bob Blaines, Francis Haynes's nephew, was raised on a farm

near Richmond. In 1947 at the age of seventeen, he was accidently shot in the leg while hunting. Although the nearest hospital was in Excelsior Springs, the ambulance took him to Research Hospital in Kansas City for surgery. After the surgeon amputated his leg, he left the end open to drain and told him to return to the hospital in two weeks, when the surgeon would sew the wound edges together. It healed without infection. Bob Blaines benefited from a lesson learned by surgeons in the war; delayed closure of dirty or contaminated wounds saved lives. Today he would have had removal of dead tissue, maybe a blood-vessel graft, using either a piece of vein from his good leg or a tube made from a nylonlike cloth, and probably escaped amputation of his leg. Similarly, Francis Haynes would have had the blood vessels repaired or, if possible, the arm sewn back on by repairing of the nerves, blood vessels, and muscles.

Missouri medicine became internationally recognized in 1944 when the Nobel committee awarded Dr. Joseph Erlanger and Dr. Herbert Gasser of Washington University the Nobel Prize in medicine. In 1947 Carl F. and Gerty T. Cori shared another Nobel Prize in physiology of medicine for their discovery of how glycogen, a starchlike substance stored in the liver and muscle, is converted to sugar in the body for energy. In all, Washington University proudly claims fifteen Nobel laureates who carried out their research at that institution or received some of their research training there.

Sporadic cases of poliomyelitis (polio) had occurred before 1943, but that summer a severe epidemic made Missouri parents keep their children away from swimming pools, movie theaters, or anyplace where crowds could be expected. In the *Journal of the American Medical Association* in 1947, Dr. Albert B. Sabin of Cincinnati, the discoverer of the first polio vaccine, wrote: "peculiar circumstances which may contain an important clue is that epidemics have occurred with greatest frequency and severity in the very countries in which sanitation and hygiene have undoubtedly made their greatest advances." Dr. Sabin's statement must have added to the terror of that summer as parents realized that the progress made in health care could not shield their children from the danger of polio.

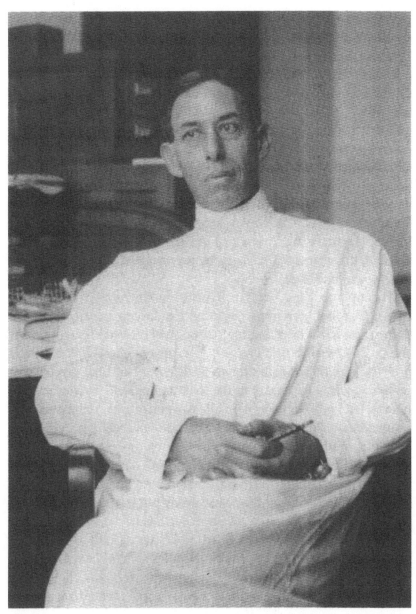

Dr. Joseph Erlanger received the Nobel Prize in Medicine in 1944, along with his colleague Dr. Herbert Gasser, for research on nerve impulses. (Bernard Becker Medical Library, Washington University School of Medicine in St. Louis)

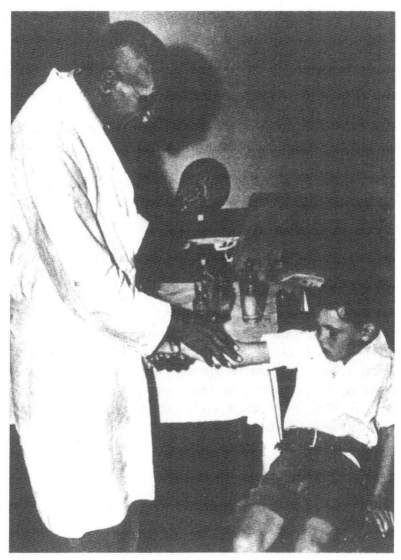

George Washington Carver, a great American agronomist, was born in a cabin near Joplin and lived there for twelve years. Shown here in 1937, he massages the arm of a boy with infantile paralysis at the Tuskegee Institute, where he became world famous for his numerous contributions in the use of farm crops, especially products made from peanuts. The George Washington Carver National Monument and a park are located just off Interstate 44 near Joplin. (Tuskegee Institute, Tuskegee, Alabama, courtesy State Historical Society of Missouri, Columbia)

Another observation by scientists created further mystery. They noticed that the majority of patients who were paralyzed by the disease were older than before. In 1916, most of those paralyzed (95 percent) had been younger than ten; in 1947, only 52 percent were young children.

Hospitals established wards with "iron lungs"—huge tanks that enclosed all but the heads of patients with high-level paralysis. Changing pressure in the tanks substituted for the patients' breathing. Physical therapy departments expanded to rehabilitate as much as possible those victims with limb weakness and paralysis, and scientists developed more sophisticated breathing machines.

Polio vaccination programs spread throughout Missouri. In 1954, 9,500 second graders in the state had received three injections. In the spring and summer of 1955, an additional 150,000 received one or two injections. The vaccine worked; there were only 265 cases of polio in Missouri in 1955, the smallest number since the years before the epidemic of 1943.

Winning against the scourge of polio had set the stage for the miraculous advances of the next fifty years. Blood transfusions, antibiotics, and vaccinations against childhood diseases would completely change health care. Easter Seal posters and iron lungs would give way to the attack on the diseases known as the big three: heart disease, stroke, and cancer.

Part IV
Scientific Medicine
1949–1999

Two of the most important scientific advances after the 1950s were the advances in imaging technology and the ability to modify the rejection process in organ transplantation.

—C. Rollins Hanlon, 1997

Introduction

By 1949 the United States had recovered from World War II and entered a period of unmatched prosperity. In 1956 Congress passed the Federal Interstate Highway and Defense Act. With the advent of the interstate system and the connecting state highways, cars and trucks overshadowed trains as methods of transportation. Although railcars still moved many goods, railroad stations went the way of river towns: the highway system relegated Union Station in Kansas City and in St. Louis as well as smaller stations throughout Missouri to monuments of a previous era. The airplane industry grew rapidly, and Missouri had a large part of the growth. The public liked speed, and airplanes now transported passengers and goods. The new ways of traveling and shipping seemed to threaten the railroads' very survival.

As before, faster and more frequent travel meant new kinds of medical care were required. Epidemics followed travelers. The Hong Kong flu epidemic of 1957 made it from China to most major cities in the United States within days. Missouri, like other states, was only one day removed from epidemics anywhere in the world. On the positive side, medical advances anywhere in the world were only one day away from Missouri.

Rapid world travel ultimately brought goods from every part of the globe to the United States, and with it an old environmental problem recurred. In 1996, 9,000 people died in the U.S. from food poisoning. *E. coli*, a common pathogen in feces, caused most of these deaths, and investigators traced the source to foreign imports from countries where the tomatoes, strawberries, or other fruit had been irrigated with wastewater. The deaths served as a stark reminder that the water and food supply must be monitored continually.

Medical advances in the last decades of the twentieth century led to an understanding of immunity, the way the body resists and rejects implants of any foreign material or tissue, so-called natural immunity. Many Missourians had developed some understanding of immunity through observation. Gus Reid was born early in the twentieth century and grew up in Des Moines. She recalls,

> The old folks always warned about "the dread of the second summer of childhood. Babies had immunity from the mother's milk for six or nine months. So in the next summer when they were old enough to be taken around town, they were exposed to the bacterial and viral infections going around. And they ate store food and got unpasteurized milk in place of mother's milk.

A new and unexpected problem also arose: money for medical services ran out, and the era proved one of Mark Twain's sayings, "The lack of money is the root of all evil." Accelerating health costs and decreasing reimbursement forced a change in old-fashioned medical criteria for hospitalizations, as well encouraging shorter hospital stays. Fewer admissions and shorter stays in the hospital decreased the demand for nurses. Tighter budgets further affected nursing, as less expensive and less qualified caregivers replaced nurses.

Scientific advances made possible new medical treatments, but some of those flew in the face of religious beliefs, breaking open the old wounds between religion and science and creating ethical problems. Conflict over theory and teachings in prior eras had erupted into warfare, and now medicine was ready to move beyond argument into action.

10

Viruses and Chemicals
Everywhere

Compared to previous periods, the environment of the last fifty years has presented numerous and complex threats to health. No longer do acute ailments such as cholera, typhoid, or smallpox pose a threat. Flu epidemics that spread rapidly by air travel around the world do not claim as many victims. With potent antibiotics available, the complication that killed flu patients in previous eras, pneumonia, strikes mainly the infirm. Although there are several minor outbreaks of upper respiratory or gastrointestinal viral ailments every year, annual vaccinations, administered to the elderly and those with chronic medical problems, reduces their number and severity.

But pollution of streams and ground by industrial waste has grown along with industry. Efforts to control air pollution by regulating emissions from factories and from automobiles have spawned new enterprises. This form of environmental contamination is easy to monitor, and its harmful effects on health are immediate and measurable. By studying the increase of visits to emergency rooms and physicians offices for complaints about breathing problems, such as asthma, bronchitis, or emphysema, health officials can readily measure the effects and amounts of pollution.

Accidents that result in contamination of the environment are also easy to detect. In 1979 a railroad tanker car spilled chemicals in Sturgeon, Missouri. Claims of illness from chemical toxicity grew, and the resultant lawsuit went on for years, mostly because a scientific connection between illness and exposure to chemical fumes could not be proven.

Determining the extent of contamination of soil from toxic

chemical waste proves an even more difficult problem. The frightening results of Agent Orange used in Vietnam served as a wake-up call to Missouri. Investigators found dioxin, the cancer-producing chemical attributed to many ailments suffered by the veterans of the Vietnam War, in the soil in Times Beach. Supposedly, the road oil used in asphalt streets contained the chemical. The federal government relocated the occupants of Times Beach, creating a ghost town. In June 1997 as workers burned the last bit of contaminated soil, reports suggested the dioxin levels in the soil at Times Beach had not posed a threat to the citizens. Since then the Department of Natural Resources has developed a "Route 66 Park" at Times Beach.

Major natural disasters during the last half of the twentieth century were few. Minor rumblings along the New Madrid fault reminded the citizens of the "big one," the earthquakes of 1811–1812, and the bigger one expected by experts. Local flooding occurred several times, but the great flood of 1993 covered the floodplain of the Mississippi River and spread out along the entire stretch of the Missouri River through the state. While the flooding defied man and his levee system, surprisingly, it caused few problems in health, a tribute to the control of waste and water supplies.

As it had with World Wars I and II, medicine used lessons learned from experience in the Korean and Vietnam Wars. Two lessons, efficient handling of mass casualties and care of the severely injured in emergency rooms, designated trauma centers, saved lives. The American College of Surgeons formed state trauma committees. The Missouri Chapter, chartered in 1976, set up standards for the care of injuries. To receive the severest injuries, an emergency room needed to have trained trauma physicians in the hospital twenty-four hours a day. The legislature required that ambulances have certified emergency medical trained personnel as well. During the Korean War, helicopters were used to take wounded soldiers from the field to the hospital. Dr. Frank Mitchell, professor of surgery at the University of Missouri–Columbia and chairman of the Trauma Committee for Missouri since 1976, initiated their use in Missouri.

"Helicopters came into use in the late 70s. At first we used the

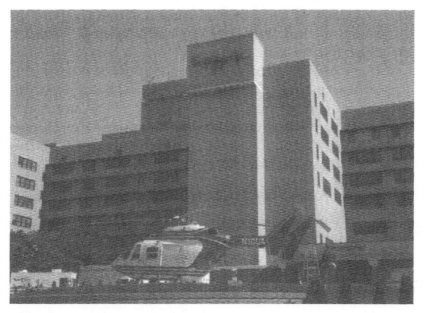

Helicopter on helipad in front of the emergency room of the
University Hospital. (photo by the author)

highway patrol chopper. The university acquired a helicopter in
1982, and by 1997 it had made over 15,000 runs," he said. The
only crash occurred early in the program when the engine failed,
but fortunately, no one died as a result. A medical evacuation program by helicopter soon followed in St. Louis and Kansas City
and grew to eleven programs in Missouri by 1997. Personnel care-
fully monitor flights for necessity and effectiveness.

Dr. Mitchell kept records on the value of the helicopter for medical emergencies. "We reviewed our data and found that, after the
fact, analysis of detailed medical findings indicated that in 15 percent
of the cases the helicopter was not absolutely needed. But 25 percent
of those who were rushed to our trauma center by chopper and survived would have died en-route if transported by ambulance."

On July 17, 1981, the Hyatt Hotel tragedy, the largest death toll
from a hotel disaster in the United States, killed 113 people and
injured 188 others when a walkway collapsed due to a structural

defect. Kansas City had a medical disaster plan, a legacy of the Korean and Vietnam Wars, and had tested hospitals' readiness with annual disaster drills.

Without trained paramedics and a well-established disaster plan, many of the people injured would have died. On July 22 the *Kansas City Star* interviewed some of the rescuers. "Firefighter Harold Knabe described how a rescuer heard the moans of an 11-year-old boy about five hours after the collapse. A firefighter, Michael Trader, [stayed] on his belly for more than an hour talking to him and reassuring him while we went to work with jackhammers and blowtorches." They pulled out first the eleven-year-old and then his mother. The boy had minor injuries. His mother, Connie Downing, had serious injuries: a broken ankle, a broken pelvis, internal injuries, and significant facial injuries. She and her son were the next-to-last victims to be removed alive. After a lengthy rehabilitation, Mrs. Downing went back to school, got a master's degree in nursing, and taught at Kansas University Medical Center. Twenty-six years later she remembers the bravery and dedication of the rescuers. "We had been buried all night long . . . a little firefighter [got] on his belly and talked to my son for hours. Sometime early in the morning my son asked, 'Mommie, are we going to die?' I told him, 'We probably are but it's better than where we are now.'"

As people began to move from the cities to the suburbs, Missouri faced huge new environmental health hazards. For years, the legislative bodies, state and local, had wrestled with the problem of physician distribution. Physicians had joined rural citizens in moving to cities. When large cities became crowded, people began to leave for the suburbs. Doctors and most hospitals moved to the growing suburban areas, leaving a core of old structures to serve the poor who stayed in the cities. In the inner cities enemies to health grew that dwarfed the chronic health demons, tobacco and alcohol abuse. Drug abuse increased to seeming epidemic proportions and then spread to the suburbs. Violence spread, creating unheard-of challenges for medicine. Drug problems, though not new to emergency rooms, meant increased numbers of stabbing and shooting victims. Crack babies were born in increasing numbers, and stubborn addictions developed in adults. Legislatures and medical organizations tried plan after plan without success.

During this time, new drugs became available for patients who had been confined in mental hospitals. Many patients were released from institutions. In the 1990s, the number of people hospitalized was only about 100,000, one-sixth of what it had been in the 1950s. Released patients often had no place to go, and many went to live in the inner cities—often on the streets. Twenty-seven percent of the homeless came from institutions, joining those who chose homelessness as well as those who were forced into it. Residents of inner cities ran greater health risks than those who lived in other parts of the state in spite of social efforts, regulations, and the spending of millions of dollars trying to solve the problems. Soon, the environmental dangers reached past cities to the suburbs and then to small towns.

Despite the problems created for some patients released from institutions under drug therapy, many patients benefited from drugs that controlled epilepsy or certain mental problems. With medication, not only could patients be released from "colonies" for those with epilepsy, homes for the mentally disturbed, and various kinds of hospitals, but many could find jobs and become productive citizens.

Routine immunization of infants and children practically eliminated childhood diseases. Fifteen hundred cases of diphtheria per 100,000 people struck the U.S. in 1920, but in 1970, only a small number of cases occurred—0.05 per 100,000. Smallpox struck 111,672 people in 1920, but after 1950 authorities reported no cases. In 1960, before the introduction of measles vaccine, there were 441,703 cases of the disease (a rate of 245.4 per 100,000), and 380 died of it. In 1984, there were only 2,586 cases (1.1 per 100,000), and only 1 person died. Whooping cough caused only ten deaths in 1990. Besides virtually eliminating many contagious diseases in children, vaccines also protected many adults from the diseases that had killed so many in previous years.

With the old lethal diseases controlled, this modern environment was fertile soil for new health problems from the viruses, for which there were no miracle curative antibiotics or vaccines. Hepatitis viruses contaminated the blood supply, and, from time to time, the food supply. Medicine responded as it had with epidemics of the past, such as cholera, by quarantining "sources" of the contamination and requiring mandatory testing (i.e., blood donors and food handlers). The methods were successful, and the threat was greatly reduced.

Not so with the AIDS virus, the cause of "acquired immunodeficiency disease." Transmitted by sexual contact and by contaminated needles, it threatened the blood supply and inspired a panic similar to that seen with the polio epidemic of the 1940s. However AIDS has been handled differently. Carriers of the virus have not been quarantined or isolated. Civil rights laws made mandatory testing illegal. Unlike in previous eras, when public health laws required the isolation of patients with diseases such as tuberculosis, cholera, measles, diphtheria, or others for which no treatment existed, no laws restricted patients who tested positive for the AIDS virus. Thus a nurse with AIDS could continue drawing blood or giving injections to patients. Officials reported 125 cases of AIDS in the U.S. from 1971 to 1981. From 1981 through 1994 a total of 435,319 adults and adolescents developed AIDS, and 267,479 (61 percent) died.

Community health problems created by absent or defective sewage systems that contaminated the water or food supply and epidemics such as poliomyelitis became less common. Wars became primarily local or regional conflicts. Medicine, through government regulations and advances in science, had decreased health hazards and increased longevity for the people of Missouri. But science and social disasters led to new challenges for the second half of the century. Missourians were affected by new environmental risks to health; some sprang from scientific advances and others were created by social behavior and lifestyles. Officials labeled the expense of caring for any and all of these problems a "health cost."

11

Specialization and Immunization

Medicine entered the second half of the twentieth century with a strong foundation. State and local governments had established firm guidelines for eliminating or controlling environmental factors that put health at risk and, in cooperation with the state medical association, set down qualifications for excellence in health care from medical education, to physician licensing, to hospital certification.

The industrial and scientific revolution after World War II had brought medical advances that created a huge demand for medical personnel. Sophisticated technology required trained specialists. Most specialty boards had been established before World War II: the American Board of Obstetrics and Gynecology was formed in 1927, the American Board of Internal Medicine in 1936, and the American Board of Surgery in 1937. Operation of high-tech equipment and performance of highly sophisticated procedures required specially trained physicians.

This proved true for nursing as well. In addition to fulfilling the traditional role of compassionate caregiver, the nurse with a college degree could acquire a master's or Ph.D. and become a team manager. Nurse midwife, nurse anesthetist, operating room nurse, nurse clinician, and other specializations catapulted nursing into the center of the medical scientific revolution. Nursing programs grew rapidly to fill the demand. As professional groups for physicians had done, nursing organizations grew in sophistication and influence. Nursing leaders formed the American Association of College of Nurses in 1969 and the American Academy of Nurses in 1973. By 1975, 35 programs that offered basic education in professional nursing were in Missouri, and 15,257 regular nurses worked full-time or part-time in the state.

Major changes occurred in medical education in Missouri in the

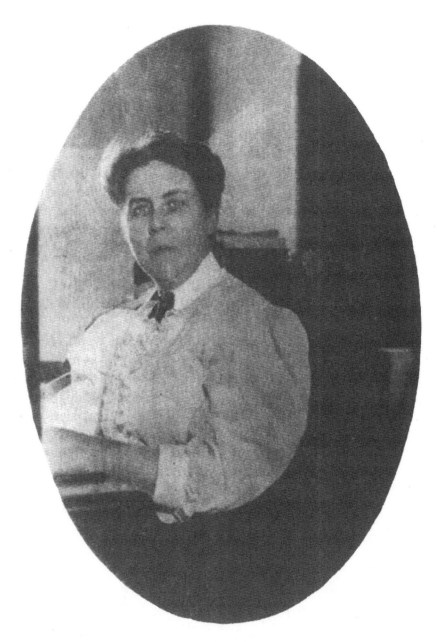

Gertrude M. Gibson of St. Louis, first president of the Missouri State
Nurses Association. (State Historical Society of Missouri, Columbia)

last half of the century. More women entered medical schools after the war. Women had made up less then 5 percent of the students at the University of Missouri–Columbia in 1930. Ten percent of the entering medical students in 1960 and 60 percent in 1990 were women. Before World War II fewer than 10 percent of medical school faculty members were female. By 1985 women made up 17.7 percent nationwide.

Dr. Elizabeth James, professor of pediatrics at the University of Missouri Medical School in Columbia, remembers the hardships she faced during her studies in the postwar era. She entered the medical school in 1965, one of two female students out of a class of eighty-five. As a junior she took night call on the hospital wards, requiring her to remain in the hospital all night. But no sleeping rooms for female students or female residents on call existed. "If I got a chance to sleep, I generally slept in the ward chart room with my head on folded arms. Sometimes a nurse would cover my shoulders with a blanket. A few times a nurse found an empty bed and I got a great night's sleep."

The University of Missouri's role in medical training has undergone many changes since then. In 1953 it moved to a four-year program in Columbia. And in 1969 Governor Hearnes signed a bill that provided $150,000 toward planning a new medical school to be located in Kansas City. Directed by Dr. E. Grey Dimond, who had returned to Kansas City as provost for health sciences and distinguished professor of medicine at the University of Missouri School of Medicine at Kansas City in 1968, Missouri's new medical school admitted eighteen students in 1970; in 1977 it graduated forty-four.

UMKC medical school had several features different from the traditional four-year medical school, which requires three or four years of premedical training. The dream of Dr. Dimond was to develop a school with six years combined premedical-medical training and to accept students directly from high school. A faculty of specially oriented teachers, called docents, instructed students.

The venture proved successful; graduates of UMKC fared well on examinations and obtained specialty training spots, performing along with students from traditional programs. When asked why

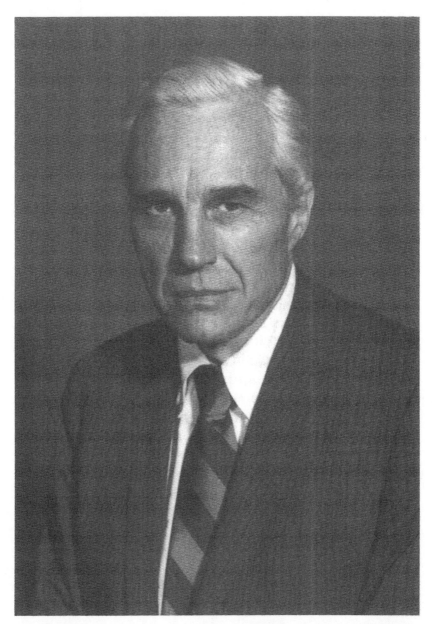

Dr. E. Grey Dimond was born in St. Louis and graduated from Indiana Medical School. From 1950 to 1960 he served as professor and chairman of the Kansas University Medical School's department of medicine, while maintaining a cardiovascular research laboratory. (courtesy Dr. Dimond)

students attended only six years rather than eight with separate premedical and medical courses, Dr. Dimond responded, "Mainly because I went through medical school in the accelerated army program during the war and found that those who went through it made perfectly good doctors . . . if you're training to be a professional, why have three months off in the summer? . . . so we gave up the usual holidays and vacation time."

After World War II the economics of medical care changed. Payment for doctors' visits and hospitalization shifted from patients to insurance carriers, expanding until insurance covered outpatient care as well. "If the patient couldn't pay, I took a chicken or a sack of potatoes," wrote Dr. Saugrain in the early 1800s. "Before health insurance became popular, things weren't much different in Maryville," said Dr. Elvin C. Imes. "In the early fifties a patient couldn't pay for his operation so he gave me a case of strawberries." Dr. Imes had finished the two years of medical school then offered by the university and graduated from the University of Louisville School of Medicine. He began practice in Ridgeway with Dr. Lane Brewer, the eighth female to graduate from the Missouri School of Medicine. Dr. Brewer had graduated in 1908, two years before the school reverted to a two-year program, granting a Master of Science in medicine.

Until the 1960s physicians and hospitals treated people who were unable to pay as a matter of course. When the population began to shift from rural to urban areas in search of jobs, it created pressures on this philosophy of care. The inner city had inexpensive housing and residents who needed free care. Large city-county hospitals were built to provide that care. The most noted, St. Louis City Hospital, the Homer G. Phillips Hospital for Afro-Americans in St. Louis, and Kansas City General Hospital grew, requiring more and more city, county, and state tax dollars for support. Health care at these facilities could not equal that at private hospitals for a number of reasons.

Problems common in the decaying cores of cities—alcoholism, violence, drugs, and poverty—led to medical complications that cost a great deal to treat. Demand soon exceeded resources. Studies showed that multiple factors contributed to poorer health care for the inner city. While many inner-city health facilities were underfunded, delay in diagnosis seemed to play a large role in lower survival rates for many conditions, such as cancer, heart disease, and strokes. Also, some patients could not understand or follow the treatment plan or get checkups because of poor education, limited resources, and lack of transportation.

In July 1965, President Lyndon Johnson came to President Harry Truman's home in Independence to sign the Medicare Act, which provided federal health insurance for citizens over sixty-five. At the last moment, Congress had appended the Medicaid provisions to the act, producing a bill that would irrevocably change medical care. Thus Missourians over sixty-five as well as citizens with disabilities, the indigent, or those with incomes below the poverty level became eligible for health care at private physicians' offices and private hospitals. While this law reflected the philosophy of its supporters, quality health care regardless of ability to pay, an immediate negative effect was to be seen on the inner-city hospitals of the state. With Medicare and Medicaid programs in place, the city, county, and state charity hospitals lost many of their patients. St. Louis City Hospital closed its doors in 1973, and plagued by low numbers of patients, Kansas City General Hospital, in need of major repairs, closed and fell to the wrecking ball. Truman Medical Center, a smaller, modern facility constructed across the street from the old hospital, replaced it.

Medicare and Medicaid programs affected Ellis Fischel Hospital as well. It became the hospital for the poor who had cancer and did not qualify for Medicare or Medicaid. Wendy Evans has worked at Ellis Fischel for twenty-seven years, first as a staff nurse and now, with a master's degree, as associate director of the hospital. She remembers, "Not only did the census drop after medicare and medicaid, but those that were finally sent to us were at a more advanced stage."

When it was taken over by the University of Missouri Medical School at Columbia, Ellis Fischel's potential for revival seemed real. "Since the merger in 1990, our numbers have increased . . . private doctors join university physicians in giving multidisciplinary care . . . and we now have a reputation as a good cancer center for private patients," Evans says.

The Veterans Health Administration, established by the United States Congress in 1936, made little impact until after 1950. The Veterans Administration Hospital in Kansas City opened in 1949 and became aligned with the University of Kansas School of Medicine, a marriage that could not be broken when the University of Missouri opened its medical school in Kansas City, Missouri. Other VA hospitals opened in the early 1950s, one in Poplar Bluff in 1951 and another in St. Louis in 1952 as the John Cochran Veterans Administration Hospital. At the six outpatient facilities around the state, veterans from both world wars and the Korean, Vietnam, and Gulf Wars can receive free care in some cases.

The lack of adequate financial support for the Veterans Hospitals in Missouri, and for the other 170 in the U.S., has proven to be a problem, as use strains capacity. The Veterans Administration Hospital in Columbia opened in 1973. It is affiliated with the University of Missouri. By affiliating, VA hospitals share doctors, the patients are available for teaching and training students and residents, and the university hospital performs specialized tests and procedures not available in VA facilities. When the VA Hospital in Kansas City affiliated with the University of Kansas Medical Center and the St. Louis VA Hospital affiliated with Washington University Medical Center and St. Louis University Medical School, highly trained faculty was available to the system. This brought more patients to the medical school. It also helped the VA hospitals, which in the early days had been criticized for giving below-standard care because of the difficulty in hiring excellent physicians.

12

New Parts

World War II had imposed restrictions and hardships on those at home as well as those in the armed services. Rationing meant shortages of gasoline, tires, sugar, and other manufactured goods. The end of the war brought relief from rationing. And lessons learned in war brought advances in medical treatment. One of the earliest successes based on experiences of the war was the lens implant. Physicians had noted that eye injuries caused by the plastic used in cockpit canopies created little if any inflammatory reaction. Physicians experimented with plastic lens implants after removal of cataracts in the Netherlands and England at the end of the 1940s, and the procedure became common in the 1950s. Dr. Robert C. Drews of St. Louis recalls he was the first to implant the modern version.

In the fall of 1996, Shirley Drummond of Columbia went to the hospital and under local anesthesia had cataracts removed and a new lens implanted in each eye. "The next day I went to the doctor's office and they removed the patch. I could see perfectly and I didn't even have stitches . . . and no coke bottle glasses."

In the 1950s, the heart-lung machine was developed. It was used for open-heart surgery and made it possible to replace patients' heart valves scarred from rheumatic fever. For some patients, the scarring was mild, but for others it grew worse over time and prevented the heart from working well. During open-heart surgery, surgeons removed the scarred heart valve and sewed a metallic one in place.

In 1956 Dr. C. Rollins Hanlon of St. Louis University did the first open-heart operation in Missouri. Dr. Hanlon received his M.D. from Johns Hopkins and interned there. He went to Cincinnati for residency and became chairman of surgery at St. Louis University in 1950. "Washington University's heart team

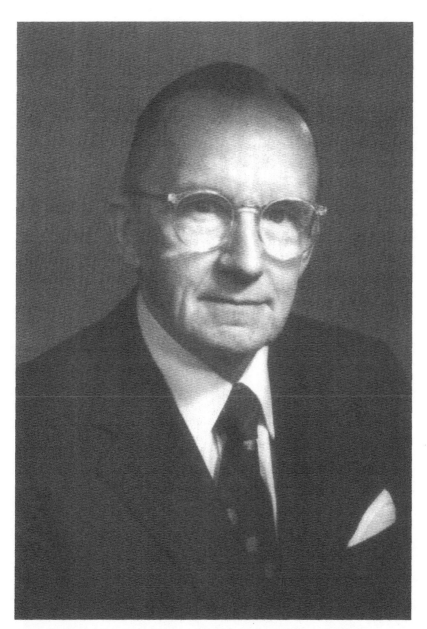

Dr. C. Rollins Hanlon performed the first open-heart operation in Missouri in 1956. Beginning in 1969, he served as director of the 25,000–member American College of Surgeons. (courtesy Dr. Hanlon)

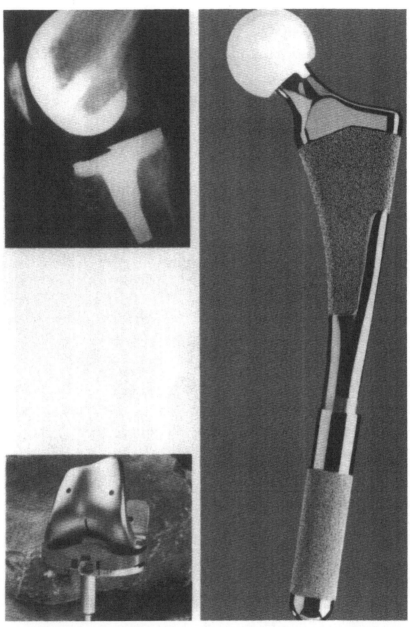

Implants for worn-out joints: Upper left, x-ray of knee implant in place; lower left, frontal view of knee implant; right, the implant used for a new hip. (courtesy Larry Gross, Columbia, and Smith and Nephew Orthopedics, Memphis)

joined in the battle to fix diseased heart valves two years after we did our first," he said with a chuckle.

Removable metallic objects had been tried before permanent ones came into use; metal plates in the head and metal rods in the thigh bone after fractures had been successful. Before long surgeons routinely performed total hip and total knee replacements, taking out the bad joints and inserting implants, rescuing patients from pain and restricted activities.

Medicine took another giant leap forward when Dr. Joseph Murray in Boston performed the first kidney transplant in 1956. The body reacted strongly to reject another person's kidney, even when the donor's tissue had been chosen because it matched the recipient's. With weak drugs to suppress the patient's immune system, the earliest transplants succeeded only about half the time.

Dr. Bill Newton performed the first kidney transplant in Missouri in 1958. The surgery was a joint effort of Washington University and St. Louis University, and Newton performed the procedure at the John Cochran VA Hospital in St. Louis. Drugs to suppress the immune system had improved by the time Dr. Gilbert Ross performed his first kidney transplant on Ed Meyer at the University of Missouri–Columbia, on February 11, 1972. By 1997 his team had performed six hundred. Patients escaped kidney dialysis, which required a weekly trip to the hospital, where the patient's blood was passed through a machine that removed the waste products normally removed by good kidneys. In addition to the ordeal of weekly needle-sticks, the patient slowly lost weight and grew sicker.

The remarkable thing about implants is that not only do they save lives but they allow recipients to go back to living normally, although many patients still must take daily medication. Brad Ford received a kidney from his mother in 1988 and still takes several drugs every day to keep his body from rejecting it. He is a golf professional at the Country Club of Missouri in Columbia. I asked him what the kidney transplant meant for him. "Life," he said and lined up the next putt.

Dr. Vallee Willman and Dr. George Kaiser performed the first heart transplant in Missouri in 1972 at St. Louis University, and

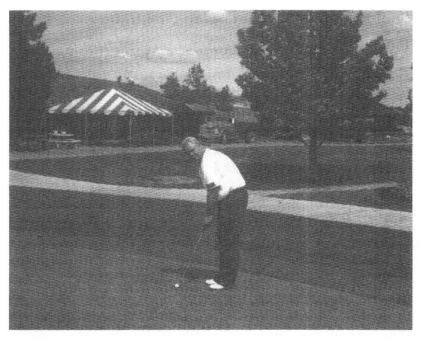

Brad Ford, club professional at the Country Club of Missouri, Columbia, eight years after receiving a kidney transplant. (photo by the author)

Dr. Thomas Helling performed the first liver transplant in Missouri at St. Luke's Hospital in Kansas City in 1980. In both cases, drugs again had to be used to stop the patients' immune systems from attacking the new organs.

However, blocking the immune system causes problems. A patient can die of infection because the drugs prevent his or her body from fighting it. That danger forced doctors to move slowly in trying to transplant other organs. But when a new drug, Cyclosporine, became available as an experimental drug in 1981, transplantation vaulted forward. Cyclosporine prevented the white blood cells (called T-lymphocytes) responsible for rejecting the graft (or transplanted organ) from reproducing or maturing. With the new drug, both doctors and patients were ready for new heart and new liver transplants. Rejection rates had been very high, but by the mid-1980s, graft survival had improved 10 to 30 percent.

Pharmacologic research produced new drugs, many alleviating, controlling, or curing diseases. Before their use, many of the diseases required repeated operations, some major procedures, in an attempt to relieve symptoms or prolong life. As in previous eras, new technology brought with it new medical problems. Hepatitis from blood and its products as well as from contaminated needles began to spread, and new regulations were needed to control production and use of all products administered through the bloodstream.

Scientific medicine changed the face of most specialties with another gigantic step, new imaging techniques. The radiologist, an interpreter of shadows on the x-ray film that revealed clues of some ailments, became a highly trained physicist and a hands-on diagnostician. For fifty years physicians used radiopaque material, giving it to patients to swallow in the form of barium to demonstrate the presence of stomach ulcers, or injecting it as a radiopaque solution into the spinal fluid to visualize a disc or other abnormalities causing problems. Then angiography, the injection of radiopaque dyes in arteries to visualize abnormalities, opened exciting new horizons for medicine. Computerized axial tomography, the CAT scan, can look inside body cavities, the skull, spine, or joints and reveal abnormalities, saving patients the expense and pain of exploratory surgery. Magnetic resonance imaging, MRI, permits the same advantage without exposing the patient to radiation. PET scans, positron emission tomography, use an imaging technique that reveals the function of organs; for example, they reveal the biochemical activity of the brain. These procedures, performed by million-dollar machines and highly skilled technicians and specialists, surpass the cost of many operations, but prevent many painful and unnecessary surgical procedures, make many diagnoses possible sooner, and reveal problems previously relegated to guesswork or at best "clinical impression."

Just as infection following a gunshot wound was the greatest cause of fear during the Civil War, so infection after placing a foreign object, an implant, in the body also caused fear. To a great extent, research has quieted those fears by developing new, powerful antibiotics. From implantable, permanent teeth, to implantable pacemakers to regulate heartbeat, to artificial hips, knees, shoulders, fingers, and toes, the use of implants to replace worn-out or damaged human parts became commonplace. Implants did not replace plants with powers to cure used in earlier medical treatment. Instead, they required more of them to ward off rejections and infections.

Further scientific advances have changed several commonly performed operations. When a patient has a clogged artery, the cardiologist, or heart doctor, passes a small tube in the artery to the leg or the heart and opens up narrow areas, sparing many patients major operations. Laparoscopic surgery, performed through small incisions made in the belly wall as an outpatient procedure, is common for operations on the gallbladder, hernia repairs, and some stomach operations.

Advances in medicine have raised the expected survival for Missourians; at the beginning of the twenty-first century, citizens can expect to live about seventy-eight years. With childhood diseases, polio, tuberculosis, and most contagious diseases eliminated almost a half century ago, the assault on organ diseases produced striking results for several ailments.

Yet, in 1996 according to an independent study carried out by the Morgan Quinto Corporation, Missouri was "the 43rd healthiest state . . . ranked second only to Indiana for the largest percentage of overweight adults . . . also had the second highest death rate behind West Virginia."

A study of changes in death rates from certain diseases sheds light on part of the problem.

Table 7 shows a striking decrease in death rates for tuberculosis and a modest decrease in deaths from motor vehicle accidents and strokes. But cancer deaths increased significantly, as did death from heart attacks caused by blockage of arteries to the heart. From 1940 to 1961, deaths from kidney disease and inflammations (which includes pneumonia) decreased dramatically and

Table 7. *Death Rate per 100,000 Missourians*

Disease	1940	1961	1992
Diabetes	25.2	17.6	20.8
Heart disease	296.3	430.5	342.3
Stroke	99.9	89.9	67.0
Cancers	134.1	175.7	228.8
Motor vehicle	22.9	22.9	19.4
Ischemic heart	–	214.1	246.4
Pneumonia/influenza	96.0	33.7	36.5
Nephritis	112.7	8.3	11.1
Tuberculosis	46.5	5.9	0.5
All causes	1024.2	811.8*	980.0

* This figure is for 1960.

Sources: Statistical Abstracts of the United States, 1942 and Missouri Division of Health Statistical Services, Missouri Public Health Statistics: Vital Statistics, 1962, 1992

then, along with the cardiovascular and renal death group, increased from 1961 to 1992. This reversal requires investigation.

Two current issues in health care demand the attention of medical professionals, hospital administrators, health insurance carriers, and legislators. The first, highlighted by the increasing number of people who are surviving to use the new medical miracles, is the rising cost of high-tech health care. Physicians offer patients the latest in drugs or operations, even when doing so means they will likely live only a few more days or weeks. Unregulated utilization has pushed tax-supported health insurance toward bankruptcy and raised premiums higher than many patients and companies with private insurance can afford.

The second, a battle for moral standards, has been less visible. Because many physicians relied solely on medical science in caring for patients, perhaps more by reflex than design, holistic medicine has grown, strengthened by the failure of science to find cures for Alzheimer's disease, cancer, and many other diseases. Also, scientific advances have sometimes conflicted with people's religious beliefs.

Joyce Marcules's reaction to illness illustrates the way many religious people have handled scientific advances. She first had cancer when she was thirty-nine. She had treatment for it, but when she was forty-three, her cancer came back. She prayed and sought care from an oncologist, a doctor who specializes in the treatment of cancer. When tests showed that the cancer was only in her liver, surgeons removed the cancer, taking 80 percent of her liver. When the cancer came back, she had more of her liver removed. Twelve years after her first operation for cancer and five years after the second liver operation, successful due to scientific advances, she said, "I believe that God wants you to use a physician and He will use the physician . . . He will guide and help you. I want to work with doctors [for health] but I want God to be in charge."

Moral and ethical concerns also surface in thinking about transplantation. Demand for organs forces people to ask questions like, "When is the brain dead so we can harvest the kidneys?"

In 1958, in *The Pope Speaks,* Pope Pius XII said, "It remains for the doctor . . . to give a clear and precise definition of 'death' and the 'moment of death' of a patient who passes away in a state of unconsciousness." The growing use of "life support techniques" has kept the issue before the scientists and the watchful eye of theologians. Following a landmark report by a committee at Harvard Medical School, criteria emerged, and in 1981 the Missouri legislature passed a law (bill no. 1223), that set minimal standards. Dr. John Oro was an assistant professor of neurosurgery at the medical school in Columbia when in 1989 he listed specific neurologic criteria for deciding when "brain death" has occurred. Dr. Oro's conclusions were published in the Missouri State Medical Associations journal, *Missouri Medicine.* As important as the list of criteria was, Dr. Oro made a much-needed contribution in declaring, "By educating ourselves and the public that 'brain death' is death, some of the burden involved in the awkward moment of disconnecting life support machines can be erased." Dr. Oro is now chief of neurosurgery at the medical school in Columbia.

Once "brain death" has occurred, organs can be taken. But the definition of "brain death" is not always enough, as when a person is in a vegetative state but not "brain dead": they are completely unconscious with no voluntary movements, requiring nourishment through a tube placed in the stomach but needing no other device for breathing or to support blood pressure. Missourians and people all over the U.S. agonized over the Karen Quinlan tragedy that occurred April 15, 1979. She became the landmark case of the persistent vegetative state. She was in a prolonged, permanent coma not requiring life support except by tube feeding. The courts joined the battle over who had the authority to "pull the plug" or, in this case, "the tube" and stop giving her life-sustaining nourishment. The living will or advanced directive, a document in which a person explains what he or she would want to happen in such a case, is an imperfect answer. But it is a marked improvement and decisive in most cases.

At the same time that Americans questioned when life ends, they struggled over when it begins. The ability of science to manipulate life forced another serious moral controversy. With *Roe v. Wade* in 1965, abortion became available upon demand. The availability of antibiotics, blood, low complication rates, and outpatient services had made abortion safe, routine, and in demand. In Missouri the lowest number of abortions since it became legal was 4,582 in 1971 (which is 58.5 for every 1,000 live births). The highest number of abortions was performed in 1979: 29,267 (or 279.6 for every 1,000 live births). These numbers fell in 1992 to 16,240 abortions (213.7 for every 1,000 live births).

Thus many scientific advances have improved health but raised strong ethical issues. The first issue, affordability or cost of health care, involved moral problems; rationing and inability to choose one's physician or hospital, justified as necessary to reduce healthcare costs, became denial of care. While this was happening, one report revealed, some physicians got large bonuses, and some HMO administrators received six-figure salaries. Missourians were shocked, and joined by the state medical association, they demanded that the legislature fix managed care so that people using it got the best care possible. Lawmakers passed the Managed Care Reform Bill on May 14, 1997.

Hailed as one of the most comprehensive in the nation, this managed-care reform package offered numerous features that corrected problems mentioned above. Managed care organizations must disclose how much of the premium dollar goes to administration and how much to actual patient care. They must also offer members an appeals process. If the insurance company denies a course of treatment recommended by a physician, the patient can request a review of the decision. Further, they must explain the plan's benefits, preexisting condition limitations, and limitations on treatment options and referrals. These and numerous other provisions in the bill help to guarantee patients' rights.

The single most important question for the people of Missouri as they enter the twenty-first century is profound: who should have the authority to decide moral and ethical health issues for the people? Whereas medicine, health professionals, and community health agencies responded to health risks and the people's needs by offering regulations or other solutions to problems in previous times, they now answer to other agencies and carry out their demands. Differing moral opinions created an ethical crisis. People on one side of an issue often seem ready to attack people on the other, as has happened with deadly results in the abortion debate.

By looking back and appreciating past problems of health care as well as both the failed and successful attempts to solve them, the people of Missouri will be armed to understand their health needs and the ethical treatments they want in the coming century.

HEART TRANSPLANTS

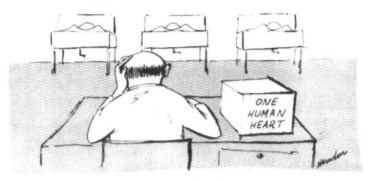

Controversy erupted when newspaper articles revealed that famous athletes or politicians received organ transplants ahead of others on the waiting list. (courtesy Orin Pederson, artist)

For More Reading

Aesculapius Was a Mizzou Tiger: History of Medicine at Ole Mizzou, by Hugh E. Stephenson, Jr., M.D. (Columbia: University of Missouri Medical School Foundation, Inc., 1998), records the history of medicine at the University of Missouri in detail with numerous illustrations.

Civil War Medicine, by Stewart Brooks (Springfield, Ill.: Charles C. Thomas Publishing Company, 1966), gives statistics of disease and battle wounds of the Civil War.

Disease in the Civil War, by Paul E. Steiner (Springfield, Ill.: Charles C. Thomas Publishing Company, 1968), describes the occurrence and deaths from disease encountered by the soldiers of the Civil War.

A Guide to the Medicinal Plants of the United States, by Arnold Krochmal and Connie Krochmal (New York: Quadrangle/New York Times Book Company, 1973), lists the plants of the United States, where they grow, and their use in medicine.

A History of Medicine in Missouri, by E. J. Goodwin, M.D. (St. Louis: W. L. Smith, 1905), describes the first physicians to arrive in Missouri, the diseases they found, and remedies they used to the end of the nineteenth century.

Medicine: A Treasury of Art and Literature, by Ann G. Carmichael and Richard M. Ratzan (New York: Hugh Lauter Levin Associates, 1991), is a synopsis of the history of medicine illustrated by beautiful photos and paintings with well-known descriptions from literature.

Medicine on the Santa Fe Trail, by Thomas B. Hall, M.D. (Arrow Rock, Mo.: Morningside Bookshop, 1971), details the diseases that afflicted travelers on the trail.

Missouri Day by Day, by Floyd C. Shoemaker (Jefferson City, Mo.: Mid-State Printing Company, 1942), tells us about changes in the environment and about people and their accomplishments as they unfolded. Physicians, institutions of higher learning, and medical schools are well done.

Missouri Folklore Society Journal, vol. 10, Donald M. Lance, general editor (Columbia, Mo.: Missouri Folklore Society, 1988). This special issue of the society journal contains sketches of two important Missouri botanists and describes the many uses of wild plants in Missouri.

Missouri's Nurses, by Edwin A. Christ (Columbia, Mo.: E. W. Stephens Publishing Company, 1957), is an accounting of the nursing movement and important nurses in the state from early times.

One Hundred Years of Medicine and Surgery in Missouri, by Max A. Goldstein (St. Louis: St. Louis Starr Publishing Company, 1900), relates the practice of medicine in Missouri's counties to the environment of the times.

One Strong Voice, by Linda Flanagan (Kansas City, Mo.: Lowell Press, 1976), records the development of nursing and the organization, education, and growth of the profession.

Washington University in St. Louis, by Ralph A. Morrow (St. Louis: Missouri Historical Society Press, 1996), has a comprehensive account of the founding and development of the university. By its in-depth consideration of surrounding events, the book enlightens us about the people in St. Louis and the rest of the state who were powerful, political, and dedicated to education.

Index